The Philosophy of Evidence-Based Medicine

To question the foundations of a discipline or a practice
is not necessarily to deny its value, but rather to stimulate a
judicious and balanced appraisal of its merits.

—R. Ashcroft & R. ter Meulen [1]

It would be difficult to put the case for the clinical trial of
new (or old) remedies more cogently or more clearly. The absence
of such a trial in the past may well have led, to give one example,
to the many years of inconclusive work on gold therapy in
tuberculosis, while...the grave dangers of much earlier and
drastic methods of therapeutics, such as blood-letting, purging,
and starvation, would quickly have been exposed by
comparative observations, impartially made.

—A.B. Hill & I.D. Hill [2]

The central problem of epistemology has always been and
still is the problem of the growth of knowledge. And the
growth of knowledge can be studied best by studying the growth
of scientific knowledge.

—Karl Popper [3]

The Philosophy of Evidence-Based Medicine

Jeremy Howick
Centre for Evidence-Based Medicine
Department of Public Health and Primary Care
University of Oxford
Oxford, UK

and

Department of Science and Technology Studies
University College London
London, UK

Foreword by Paul Glasziou

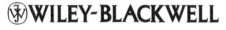

A John Wiley & Sons, Ltd., Publication

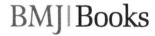

Library of Congress Cataloging-in-Publication Data

Howick, Jeremy.
The philosophy of evidence-based medicine / Jeremy Howick, with a foreword by Paul Glasziou.
    p. ; cm.
Includes bibliographical references and index.
ISBN 978-1-4051-9667-3 (pbk. : alk. paper)
  1. Evidence-based medicine. 2. Medicine—Philosophy. I. Title.
[DNLM: 1. Evidence-Based Medicine. 2. Philosophy, Medical. WB 102.5]
    R723.7.H693 2011
    610—dc22
                                                                    2010047393

A catalogue record for this book is available from the British Library.

This book is published in the following electronic formats: ePDF 9781444342659; Wiley Online Library 9781444342673; ePub 9781444342666

Set in 9.5/12pt Meridien by MPS Limited, a Macmillan Company, Chennai, India

Contents

Acknowledgments

Many of the ideas in this book about evaluating the differences between randomized trials and observational studies are John Worrall's. I am also indebted to John for extensive feedback on several chapters in the book. I am equally indebted to Nancy Cartwright and Paul Glasziou. Nancy encouraged me to write the book, and without her feedback on my chapter on mechanistic reasoning it would have been a mess. Paul, together with Jeffrey Aronson, helped me conceptualize how to combine various types of evidence and were also encyclopaedic sources of fascinating medical examples. My collaboration with Paul and Jeffrey resulted in two publications.

Most of the book was written whilst I was a Medical Research Council (MRC) funded postdoctoral research fellow (G0800055) hosted by the Centre for Evidence-Based Medicine (CEBM) at Oxford's Department of Public Health and Primary Care (DPHPC). Many people at the CEBM and DPHPC gave me invaluable advice, including Paul Montgomery, Rafael Perera, Jason Oke, Richard Stevens, Merlin Wilcox, David Mant, Amanda Burls, Alison Ward, Carl Heneghan, Su-May Liew, and Olive Goddard. Thanks to Kay, Claire, Suzie, and Andrew for encouraging frequent tea and biscuit breaks. Sir Iain Chalmers of the James Lind Library was enormously generous with his time and enriched my work in many ways, especially by encouraging me to be succinct. On one occasion, he claimed I took 30 pages to express a message he could express in 3; I succeeded in reducing it to 15.

Concurrent with my postdoctoral fellowship at Oxford I have been teaching philosophy to medical students at University College, London (UCL). My students provided me with a platform to teach my ideas (Emily Sweetman pointed out several typos in earlier drafts), and many of my colleagues at UCL gave me useful feedback. These include Steve Miller, Josipa Petrunic, Brian Balmer, Jon Agar, Norma Morris, and especially Donald Gillies.

Many other people have listened or read the ideas in these chapters at various conferences, meetings, or email exchanges. Space doesn't permit me to mention all of them, but Gordon Guyatt, Brian Haynes, Dave Sackett, Murray and Eleanor Enkin, Alejandro Jadad, Ted Kaptchuk, Elizabeth Silver,

Eileen Munro, Jon Williamson, Federica Russo, and Beatrice Golomb (many of the ideas in the conclusion are borrowed from Dr Golomb) were all helpful. I would not have been able to write the book without (some) personal distractions, usually in the form of rowing. Thanks to Jonny Searle for making sure I woke up at 5.30 on Saturday mornings in the dark of the winter, to Paul Kelly for encouraging me to join the Wolf Pack, Colin Smith for being a recent training partner, and especially to the Great Eight (Phil, Fred, Nick, Ted, John, Sohier, Dave, Hirsh and most of all Scott Armstrong) for continuing to remind me that the world is the oyster of the bold.

Various friends, including Foad Dizadji-Bahmani, Jesse Elzinga, and Josh West, put up with me for various periods of time while I moved flats. Other friends, including Sebastien, Mark, Qarim, and Renaud, were always there when I needed them. Dick Fishlock has been a continued source of entertainment and inspiration, and Dusan gave me a break. Lastly, my mother (who I'm becoming increasingly convinced is an Angel), father (who generously supported my expensive education), sisters, Brett, John, Jack and Raven provided unconditional love that helped me keep going.

Stephen Hlophé, Mingy, and Dr Bali have helped keep me almost sane. Thank you to everyone I forgot to mention.

Foreword

In 1991 an international group formed to encourage clinicians to consider results of recent research when treating patients. They commenced writing a series of User's Guides to reading research for JAMA, the Journal of the American Medical Association, and needed a new term to signal the intention of the series. After several suggestions, the group's leader, Gordon Guyatt, proposed the term Evidence-Based Medicine. The new term was to ignite a movement that spread rapidly around the world. The methods of evidence-based medicine (EBM) have evolved since then, but the focus of the inventors – mostly clinicians – was the practical concern of bedside decision making. Understandably they paid less attention to the psychology, sociology or philosophy that might underpin EBM. However, now that EBM is well established in the medical world, deeper exploration by different disciplines seems warranted. This book is an examination and extension of the philosophy of EBM: a modern conversation between Aristotle and Hippocrates.

While the term Evidence-Based Medicine has a short history dating back to the 1990s, the ideas behind it have been evolving for centuries. A large part of the vocabulary of EBM – bias, confounding, randomization, placebo, confidence interval, etc. – has been invented and developed by statisticians and epidemiologists. But philosophers have been grappling with many of the same issues that lie behind the ideas, including the nature, and proof for, causal relationships, justification for induction, and errors in human observation, models, and reasoning. Many of these terms appear and are explained inside. Other ideas less familiar in the routine EBM books also enrich this text; for example, Phillip's paradox, nocebo effects, and probabilistic causality.

The book is a rich treasure of examples. Some are akin to zen koans: thinking about them can be a struggle but considerably deepen understanding of EBM. Consider the randomized comparison of nicotine versus placebo but where both groups were also randomised to be told they received nicotine, received placebo, or not told anything (see Figure 8.4) – a 2x3 factorial design. What do the various possible comparisons tell you? Which is better: to have the nicotine patch but be told it is placebo, or have the placebo patch but be told you received nicotine? Considering these comparisons may change the way you think about the placebo effect and the place of placebos in trials.

EBMers have been focused on teaching, and getting the evidence in practice. However, less attention has been given to the philosophical roots of EBM. In particular, we have ignored or belittled the role of mechanism. The battle between mechanists and empiricists is long standing in both philosophy and medicine, but what have the two opposing ideas to offer each other, to researchers, and to the users of research? Chapter 10 is an excellent synthesis of both camps. This chapter is a crystallization of many long afternoons of stimulating discussion between the author, Jeffrey Aronson and myself. Besides the many insights developed in those conversations and set down here, I also learned the value of having the input and insight of other disciplines on the work of EBM. And had fun in the process. The challenge of working across disciplines though is great: basic assumptions are different, purposes are different, and even the vocabulary can be different. "Proof" means different things to philosophers, doctors, detectives and distillers. But with a generous dose of good-will, we found the interdisciplinary exploration fruitful for both philosophy and medicine. And worth continuing.

This work represents an important dialogue between EBM and philosophers of science. There has been too little. I searched MEDLINE for titles which include EBM and philosophy and found only six, but all from the last 6 years. Let me end with a quote from the earliest of these articles: Ashcroft and Ter Meulen introduce a special issue of the Journal of Medical Ethics that reported on a symposium on EBM by saying: "To question the foundations of a discipline or a practice is not necessarily to deny its value, but rather to stimulate a judicious and balanced appraisal of its merits; we offer the present selection of papers in that spirit." So I hope you enjoy and learn from reading this, and seek out your local philosopher for a cup of tea or a pint of ale, and some stimulating discussion.

Professor Paul Glasziou PhD FRACGP MRCGP
Director, Department of Evidence-Based Medicine
University of Oxford, Oxford, UK

Preface

Most EBM "hierarchies" of evidence rank comparative clinical studies (including systematic reviews of randomized trials) above mechanistic reasoning ("pathophysiologic rationale") and expert judgment. Within comparative clinical studies, randomized trials are considered to offer stronger evidence than observational studies. Early EBM proponents showed that many widely used therapies that had been adopted based on "lower" forms of evidence proved to be useless or harmful when subjected to evaluation by randomized trials. In spite of the compelling rationale, the EBM philosophy of evidence leads to several paradoxes. Perhaps the most striking is that many of the treatments in whose effectiveness we have the most confidence – that we consider to be most strongly supported by evidence – have never been supported by randomized trials of any description. These treatments include automatic external defibrillation to start a stopped heart, tracheostomy to open a blocked air passage, and the Heimlich maneuver to dislodge airway obstructions. While critics have attacked various aspects of the EBM methodology, the system as a whole has, with few exceptions, escaped scrutiny. After outlining the paradoxes (Chapter 1), I investigate what EBM is (Chapter 2), and how a claim that a treatment "works" *should* be unpacked (Chapter 3). Next, I defend a method for evaluating the relative strength of comparative clinical studies (Chapter 4), and I argue that the EBM position on randomized trials is, with a slight modification, sustainable (Chapter 5). The modification is to replace categorical hierarchies that place randomized trials on top with the requirement that comparative clinical studies should reveal an effect size that outweighs the combined effect of plausible confounders. In the next three chapters I evaluate the claims that double blinding (Chapter 6) and placebo controls (Chapters 7 and 8) enhance the quality of comparative clinical studies. I then examine the EBM position on mechanistic reasoning and expert judgment (Chapters 9–11). I argue that mechanistic reasoning, while beleaguered with often unrecognized problems, should be admitted as evidence, perhaps alongside evidence from comparative clinical studies.

Meanwhile, I defend the EBM view that expert judgment is not reliable as evidence, but that expertise plays several other important roles that deserve more serious discussion in the EBM literature. My conclusion (Chapter 12) is that strict hierarchies should be replaced by the requirement that all evidence of sufficiently high quality should be admitted as evidential support, and that the various non-evidential roles of expertise deserve more discussion in the EBM literature.

PART I
Introduction

CHAPTER 1

The philosophy of evidence-based medicine

This is a thorough analysis of the justification for using evidence-based medicine (EBM) methodology. Why should we believe that EBM methods provide more reliable knowledge than other methods? While many have criticized various aspects of EBM, the system as a whole has, with a few notable exceptions [4,5], escaped careful scrutiny. One can, of course, raise critical questions about the foundations of EBM without denying its value [1]. And, in fact, my overall conclusions are mostly sympathetic with the EBM position and a central aim of this book is to clarify misunderstandings of what EBM actually involves. Much work in the philosophy of science is relevant to this analysis, including the logic of scientific discovery, the problem of underdetermination, the nature of causal inference and above all the logic of evidence (confirmation theory). Philosophers who are interested in how these central issues in the philosophy of science apply to contemporary medical science should find new and relevant material here. At the same time, medical professionals who would like to examine the underlying reasons why they should (or should not!) use EBM methods to determine whether the treatments they prescribe "work" will find this analysis useful.

1.1 What on earth was medicine based on before evidence-based medicine?

Loosely speaking, three overlapping methods for determining whether treatments are effective have competed for dominance in the history of medicine. One school has insisted that the effects of medical treatments must be

The Philosophy of Evidence-Based Medicine, First Edition. Jeremy Howick.
© 2011 Jeremy Howick. Published 2011 by Blackwell Publishing Ltd.

observed directly, usually by comparing groups of people who receive the treatment with groups who do not [6–8]. Another school has demanded that the underlying causes ("mechanisms") of health and disease must be specified before concluding that a treatment caused a cure [6,9]. In parallel with these two schools, authoritative pronouncements of clinical "experts" have often played a powerful role, sometimes trumping external evidence. The EBM movement recently weighed in heavily on the side of the first method.

With a rhetorical *tour de force*, EBM was introduced as a "new paradigm" in the early 1990s [10–12]. Less than two decades later, there are at least seven journals, a dozen books, thousands of new citations to EBM each year, and a growing number of international research centres dedicated to the practice, teaching, and dissemination of EBM. Prominent medical journals, including the *British Medical Journal*, *Journal of the American Medical Association*, and *Annals of Internal Medicine*, endorse editorial policies encouraging researchers to follow the EBM rules of evidence [13], and the *New York Times* judged EBM to be the idea of the year in 2001 [14]. EBM has also colonized other disciplines. Social scientists [15], policy-makers, and even chaplains [16] are eager to demonstrate that their practices are "evidence"-based.

But what on earth was medicine based on before 1990? Given that "evidence" simply means "grounds for belief" [17], medicine has always been evidence-based by definition. Barring cases of deliberate deception, even physicians deemed to be quacks have had grounds to believe that their therapies worked. If EBM is something new, and its proponents insist it is, it must be a specific view of what counts as (good) evidence.

The EBM "philosophy" of evidence is best expressed in the EBM "hierarchies" [18–23]. The idea behind the many different hierarchies can be summed up quite simply with three central claims (Figure 1.1).

1 Randomized trials (RCTs), or systematic reviews of many randomized trials, generally offer stronger evidential support than observational studies.

2 Comparative clinical studies in general (including both RCTs and observational studies) offer stronger evidential support than "mechanistic" reasoning ("pathophysiologic rationale") from more basic sciences.

3 Comparative clinical studies in general (including both RCTs and observational studies) offer stronger evidential support than expert clinical judgment.

Early EBM proponents showed that many widely used therapies that had been adopted based on "lower" forms of evidence proved to be useless or harmful when subjected to randomized trials. In a particularly dramatic (but not unique) example, antiarrhythmic drugs became widely used based on what was (believed to be) understood about the causes of sudden death after heart attack ("mechanistic reasoning"). However, a randomized trial

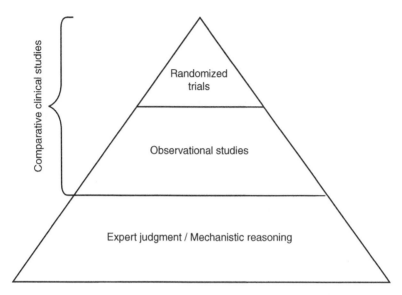

Figure 1.1 Simplified EBM hierarchy of evidence (systematic reviews of all study types is assumed to be superior to single studies).

suggested that the drugs *increased* mortality, and had killed more people every year than died in action during the whole of the Vietnam War [24]. In spite of the compelling rationale, the EBM hierarchy leads to several paradoxes. The first is that many of the treatments in whose effectiveness we have the most confidence – that we consider most strongly supported by evidence – have never been supported by randomized trials of any description. These treatments include automatic external defibrillation to start a stopped heart, tracheostomy to open a blocked air passage, the Heimlich maneuver to dislodge an obstruction in the breathing passages, rabies vaccines, penicillin for the treatment of pneumonia, and epinephrine injections to treat severe anaphylactic shock. Meanwhile we often lack confidence in some treatments that are supported by evidence from higher up the hierarchy. The antidepressant Prozac, for instance, has proven superior to placebo in some double-blind RCTs, yet the effects of Prozac (over and above "placebo" effects) are hotly disputed [25–29]. Exploiting this irony, Gordon Smith and Jill Pell wrote a spoof article entitled "Parachute use to prevent death and major trauma related to gravitational challenge: a systematic review of randomised controlled trials" [30]. They concluded that:

Advocates of evidence-based medicine have criticised the adoption of interventions evaluated by using only observational [not RCT] data.

We think that everyone might benefit if the most radical protagonists of evidence based medicine organised and participated in a double blind, randomised, placebo controlled, crossover trial of the parachute.

Strictly speaking, this critique is unfair since the EBM movement has always acknowledged that treatments with dramatic effects do not require support from randomized trials [31–34]. Yet with one recent exception [19] current hierarchies have ignored this paradox: (systematic reviews of) randomized trials still feature categorically at the pinnacle of the EBM hierarchies.

The EBM rationale for the view that comparative clinical studies provide stronger evidential support than mechanistic reasoning and clinical expertise is also problematic. While EBM proponents have always acknowledged that mechanistic reasoning is important for generalizing (see Chapter 10), and that expertise should be integrated with external evidence (see Chapter 11), the view that comparative clinical studies provide stronger evidence for efficacy than mechanistic reasoning or clinical expertise is unsupported by a defensible rationale. A stubborn objector could always claim that the conclusions from mechanistic reasoning and expert judgment were more reliable than conclusions from randomized trials. This leads to the paradox that the EBM hierarchy itself appears to be supported by "weak" (according to EBM) evidence, namely the opinion of EBM experts!

These problems suggest that although EBM is compelling on many levels, a sustained analysis is wanting. While critics have attacked various aspects of the EBM methodology, the system as a whole has, with two notable but brief exceptions [4,5], escaped scrutiny. Indeed most critics have focused on the EBM view that randomized trials are less biased than non-randomized studies [30,35–48]. While I believe there is more to say about the relative value of randomized trials, this debate is, in many ways, independent of the EBM philosophy. Bayesian philosophers of science and statisticians have been debating the relative value of randomization [49,50] since long before the EBM movement was born. More importantly, these critiques of the EBM stance on randomized trials leave the central message of EBM – that comparative clinical studies *in general* provide better evidence than mechanistic reasoning and expert judgment – untouched.

To be sure, some philosophers [5,51–56] and medical professionals [57–61] have addressed the EBM stance on "mechanistic" reasoning from the basic sciences. Yet these critiques focus on the importance of mechanistic reasoning for generalizing the results of randomized trials, a view the EBM movement has accepted since the outset [12,32–34]. The EBM view that mechanistic reasoning is inferior to comparative clinical studies for establishing that a therapy has an average clinical effect in a study population (*efficacy*) has been altogether ignored.

Similarly, while some have flagged possible problems with the EBM stance on expert judgment [62–64], and EBM proponents have proposed a model for incorporating clinical expertise [65], there have been no sustained investigations of the EBM stance on expert judgment. Indeed little critical analysis of expert judgment has been undertaken at all since the late 1970s [66].

1.2 Scope of the book

EBM raises many compelling issues that are closely linked to the question of whether their theory of evidence is acceptable. These include the practical feasibility and uptake of EBM [64,67], the supposed hijacking of EBM methodology by special interests [64,67], EBM's relationship to alternative medicine [68–70], the ethical implications of EBM [1,46,71–74], whether it is possible to adapt EBM for social science and public policy [52,72,75], how EBM can be implemented [76,77] and various other social and historical aspects of EBM [78–81].

While this book will touch on these issues in various ways, I believe it is important to analyze the EBM methodology separately for two reasons. For one, as we shall see throughout the book, many of these other problems turn on issues of strict methodology [47,74,82]. Consider, for example, the relationship between EBM and research ethics. Some accuse the EBM movement of promoting randomized trials even when we "know" that an experimental therapy is effective [46,47,83] (see Chapters 4, 7, 8 and 11). But whether or not we already know that a treatment "works" depends, to a large measure, on whether we possess sufficient supporting evidence. This, in turn, relies on our account of what counts as sufficient evidence. Hence to attack EBM on ethical grounds is parasitic on an attack of the EBM philosophy of evidence. Likewise, the relationship between EBM and alternative medicine might depend on what counts as legitimate "placebo" controls (see Chapter 7).

Then, some of these other controversies are altogether independent of the EBM philosophy. A common critique, for example, is that EBM has been hijacked by special interests. Since randomized trials are expensive, potentially profitable (i.e. patentable) treatments will be more likely to be investigated in the first place [84]. These factors are important and influence the nature and quality of research produced (see Chapter 12). If the EBM movement is serious about producing the best evidence and improving patient outcomes, its proponents should engage more actively with the powerful forces involved in producing and disseminating evidence. At the same time, special interests will attempt to influence *any* (EBM or non-EBM) methodology. Imagine for the sake of argument that the EBM philosophy was violently rejected in favor of the view that palm reading experts possessed the unassailable authority to decide whether an intervention had its putative effects. Special interests would then presumably focus on influencing palm reading experts, which could turn out to be far cheaper than conducting several large randomized trials. In brief, the problem that special interests corrupt medical research is a real problem independent of methodology. Once we address the corrupting sociological forces, we will still be left with the essential task of determining which methods most reliably detect an intervention's clinical effects.

One might argue, of course, that EBM is *particularly* prone to being hijacked by certain special interests. It is undoubtedly true, for example, that the EBM methodology is more easily used as a device to hold clinicians accountable than, say, a methodology insisting on the absolute authority of clinical experts. At the same time, if the EBM methodology is more reliable at detecting treatment effects – say it leads to saving many more lives – then the control over the medical profession allegedly attributable to EBM might be acceptable. Nobody complains that airline pilots are held accountable to a large number of rules and protocols because we believe that these rules save lives.

1.3 How the claims of EBM will be examined

Each of the three central claims of the EBM philosophy of evidence require distinct methods that I will outline separately in the relevant chapters. To summarize, I will evaluate the EBM claim that randomized trials offer superior evidential support to observational studies by appealing to the general rule that *good evidence rules out confounding factors*. Then, I will appeal to empirical evidence and analysis of relative strengths and weaknesses of mechanistic reasoning and expert judgment to evaluate the EBM claims that comparative clinical studies *generally* provide superior evidence to mechanistic reasoning and expert judgment. Contrary to what the EBM movement seem to concede, there is a strong justification for their position on the *evidential* roles of mechanistic reasoning and expert judgment.

However, there is one particular methodology that applies to the entire book and it is this: I will insist that all problems be stated clearly. With that in mind, I will spend the rest of Part I clarifying what EBM is, and what it means for a medical treatment to "work" in a clinically relevant sense. Failure to understand the nature of EBM and the nature of claims about treatment effects has led to much confusion in the critical literature.

1.4 Structure of what is to come

This book is divided into four parts. The remaining three chapters of the first part investigate what EBM is (Chapter 2) and how a claim that a treatment "works" *should* be unpacked (Chapter 3). Part II is dedicated to analyzing the EBM claim that randomized trials provide stronger evidence than observational studies, and resolving the paradox that our most effective therapies are only supported by "lower-level" comparative clinical studies. After defending a method for evaluating the relative strength of comparative clinical studies (Chapter 4), I argue that the EBM position on randomized trials is, with a slight modification, sustainable (Chapter 5). The modification involves replacing categorical hierarchies with the requirement that comparative clinical studies should reveal an effect size that is greater than the combined effect of plausible confounders. In the next three chapters I evaluate the claims that double blinding (Chapter 6) and "placebo" controls (Chapters 7 and 8) enhance the quality of randomized trials. I then introduce Part III (Chapter 9), where I examine the EBM position on mechanistic reasoning (Chapter 10) and expert judgment (Chapter 11). I argue that mechanistic reasoning, while beleaguered with often unrecognized problems, should be admitted as evidence, perhaps alongside evidence from comparative clinical studies. Meanwhile, I defend the EBM view that expert judgment is not reliable as evidence, but that expertise plays several other important roles that deserve more emphasis in discussion in the EBM literature and practice. In the conclusion (Chapter 12) I summarize the findings then point out two new classes of methodological difficulties EBM faces in the near future.

A unifying theme of the book is that ethics and epistemology are intertwined. Randomized trials are unethical if we already have sufficient evidence from observational studies (Chapter 5) or mechanistic reasoning (Chapter 9), or if we *would have* sufficient evidence had we conducted a systematic review (Chapter 2). Likewise, the debate over "placebo" versus "active" controls (Chapter 7) has important ethical implications for the approval of trials, and using expert judgment *as evidence* (judgment is required for many other roles) could be unethical if it can be proven to be harmful (Chapter 10)

By the end of the book the reader will be able to evaluate the evidence for the EBM methodology and answer the question "What is the evidence for the EBM philosophy of evidence?"

CHAPTER 2
What is EBM?

If you can believe fervently in your treatment, even though controlled tests show that it is quite useless, then your results are much better, your patients are much better, and your income is much better too. I believe this accounts for the remarkable success of some of the less gifted, but more credulous members of our profession, and also for the violent dislike of statistics and controlled tests which fashionable and successful doctors are accustomed to display.

—R. Asher [85]

The history of medicine shows many examples of forms of treatment widely considered as effective on grounds of clinical impression which have turned out to be ineffective or even harmful.

—A.B. Hill & I.D. Hill [2]

2.1 EBM as a self-proclaimed Kuhnian paradigm

The title of the paper that announced EBM to the wider community was "Evidence-based medicine: a *new* approach to teaching the practice of medicine" (my emphasis) [12]. The very first sentence of the paper reads: "A *new* paradigm for medical practice is emerging" (my emphasis) [12].

The question of whether EBM is truly new is a historical one [6,8,9,86]. While I shall provide some background to the EBM movement and recount some amusing anecdotes about early EBM advocates, a comprehensive historical analysis of the origins and genesis of EBM lies beyond the scope of this work (see Tröhler [87] for a good review of the recent historical roots of EBM). Similarly, the question of whether EBM is truly a

The Philosophy of Evidence-Based Medicine, First Edition. Jeremy Howick.
© 2011 Jeremy Howick. Published 2011 by Blackwell Publishing Ltd.

new (Kuhnian) paradigm would involve an analysis of whether Kuhnian paradigms are applicable to methodological innovations in medicine [88,89] which would take us far afield. Moreover, both questions – whether EBM is new and whether EBM is a new Kuhnian paradigm – require that we establish what EBM actually *is*. This is no straightforward task given the evolving definitions of the movement [90–93].

In this brief chapter I will contend that in spite of evolving characterizations, the EBM view that comparative clinical studies, preferably (systematic reviews of) randomized trials, provide more telling evidence for therapeutic effects than mechanistic reasoning and clinical expertise has remained constant.

I will start with a sketch of the factors that contributed to the birth of EBM movement. Then, I will review the evolving definitions of EBM and argue that its fundamental view of what counts as good *evidence* has not changed. For now, I will leave an evaluation and justifications of the EBM definition of "good" evidence for later chapters: here I will focus on charitably interpreting what the EBM system of evidence *is*.

2.2 The motivation for the birth of EBM: a sketch

The 100-year period between 1885 and 1985 brought amazing medical breakthroughs. The dramatic discovery of the rabies vaccine put an end to fear of rabid dogs, the discovery of penicillin and streptomycin suggested that infectious disease would soon be altogether eradicated, and cure for most childhood cancer was a promising sign that all cancers would soon disappear. Meanwhile, open heart surgery, hip replacements and kidney transplants indicated that we could dramatically extend our lifespans by replacing our "used" parts, and *in vitro* fertilization put an end to the misery caused by infertility [94]. Understanding the underlying *mechanisms* of health and disease appeared to drive many of these discoveries. It is difficult to see how, for example, the very idea for a rabies vaccine would have arisen without the germ theory of disease, and kidney transplants would not have been possible without understanding the immune system. The method of investigating the underlying mechanisms of disease appeared to be working well. In the century beginning in 1885 infant mortality in the USA and Europe dropped from 140 per 1000 to 5 per 1000, and life expectancy rose from under 50 to almost 80 years. It was not unreasonable to suppose, in the middle of the 20th century, that medicine would continue to advance at a furious pace and that quite soon most human suffering would all but disappear. Indeed in a 1949 article Lord Horder claimed just that: "Whither Medicine?" he asked, "Whither else than straight ahead" [95].

Eventually, however, reality set in. Infectious diseases proved more resistant than was initially envisaged, many cancers proved to be formidable opponents, and a host of ailments such as obesity, diabetes, and cardiovascular disease began to replace the traditional infectious diseases as major killers. To make things worse, the thalidomide scandal reduced the public's trust in medicine. Meanwhile, Thomas McKeown argued forcefully that increases in lifespan and decreases in infant mortality had more to do with economic improvements than medical treatments [96] and Ivan Illich, from out in left field [97], contended that medicine did more harm than good.

One thing was certain: the cost of healthcare continued (and continues) to rise each year, while improvements in healthcare (measured in life expectancy and infant mortality) have tapered off. Against this background many thoughtful clinicians began to question the value of the treatments they prescribed. Several bestselling autobiographies would be required to tell all their fascinating stories (see Daly [78] for a great overview). I will satisfy myself here with three anecdotes. Sir Iain Chalmers, who founded the Cochrane Collaboration, often tells the following story.

It was while working for a couple of years in a Palestinian refugee camp in the Gaza Strip 30 years ago that I first became aware of just how devastating a disease measles can be. We had an immunization program, supervised by the World Health Organization (WHO) staff, but measles was nonetheless common among refugee children, many of whom were malnourished and in poor health in other ways, and complications were common.

It had been drummed into me at medical school [based on mechanistic reasoning] in the early 1960s that antibiotics should never be prescribed for someone with a viral infection unless there was unambiguous evidence of bacterial superinfection. Accordingly, when a child was brought to me with early measles and I had convinced myself that there was no evidence of superinfection, I conserved our limited supply of antibiotics . . . Distressingly often, my child patients had died a few days after I had seen them.

My Palestinian medical colleague was seeing a very similar spectrum of patients with measles, but he seemed not to have a comparable experience. Toward the end of my first year working in the refugee camp, it was gently pointed out to me that this might be because he gave prophylactic antibiotics to children with measles, because, in his experience, rapid bacterial superinfection was very common in these vulnerable children. Having been convinced to change my practice, and doing exactly what I had been advised at medical school never to do, I had the impression that my child patients were less likely to die.

This clinical impression was very sobering. It made me wonder whether what I had been taught at medical school might have been lethally wrong, at least in the circumstances in which I was working, and precipitated a now incurable "scepticemia" about authoritarian therapeutic prescriptions and prescriptions unsupported by trustworthy empirical evidence [98].

Meanwhile, Dave Sackett, who was the main author on many early texts on clinical epidemiology and EBM, became unpopular even as a medical student in the 1950s for questioning the apparent wisdom of his more senior colleagues.

I was a final-year medical student on a medical ward, where a teenager with "infectious hepatitis" (now called Type A hepatitis) was admitted to my care. He presented with severe malaise, an enlarged and tender liver, and a colorful demonstration of deranged bilirubin metabolism that made me the envy of my fellow clerks. However, after a few days of total bed rest his spirits and energy returned and he asked me to let him get up and around.

In the 1950s, everybody "knew" that such patients, if they were to avoid permanent liver damage, must be kept at bed rest until their enlarged liver receded and their bilirubin and enzymes returned to normal. And if, after getting up and around, their enzymes rose again, back to bed they went. This conventional wisdom formed the basis for daily confrontations between an increasingly restless and resentful patient and an increasingly adamant and doom-predicting clinical clerk.

We clinical clerks were expected to read material relevant to the care of our patients. I wanted to understand (for both of us) how letting him out of bed would exacerbate his pathophysiology. After exhausting several unhelpful texts, I turned to the journals. PubMed was decades away, and the National Library of Medicine hadn't yet begun to help the Armed Forces Medical Library with its *Current List of the Medical Literature*. Nonetheless, it directed me to a citation in the *Journal of Clinical Investigation* (back in the days when it was a real clinical journal) for: "The treatment of acute infectious hepatitis. Controlled studies of the effects of diet, rest, and physical reconditioning on the acute course of the disease and on the incidence of relapses and residual abnormalities." (Chalmers et al. 1955). Reading this paper not only changed my treatment plan for my patient. It forever changed my attitude toward conventional wisdom, uncovered my latent iconoclasm, and inaugurated my career in what I later labeled "clinical epidemiology."

. . .Armed with this evidence, I convinced my supervisors to let me apologize to my patient and let him be up and about as much as he wished. He did, and his clinical course was uneventful.

My subsequent "clinical course" was far from uneventful. I became a "trouble-maker," constantly questioning conventional therapeutic wisdom, and offending especially the sub-specialists when they pontificated (I thought) about how I ought to be treating my patients. I had a stormy time in obstetrics, where I questioned why patients with severe pre-eclampsia received intravenous morphine until their respirations fell below 12 per minute. I gained unfavorable notoriety on the medical ward, where I challenged a consultant's recommendation that I should ignore my patient's diastolic blood pressure of 125 mmHg "because it was essential for his brain perfusion." And I deeply offended a professor of pediatrics by publicly correcting him on the number of human chromosomes (they had fallen from 48 to 46 the previous month!).

Tom Chalmers, along with Ed Fries (who answered the question about whether diastolic blood pressure should be ignored) and Archie Cochrane, became my role models. Ten years after I discharged my hepatitis patient, armed with some book learning and blessed with brilliant colleagues, I began to emulate these mentors by converting my passive skepticism into active inquiry, addressing such questions as: Why do you have to be a physician in order to provide first-contact primary care? (Sackett et al. 1974). Are the "experts" correct that teaching people with raised blood pressure all about their illness really makes them more likely to take their medicine? (Sackett et al. 1975). Just because the aorto-coronary arterial bypass is good for ischemic hearts, should we accept claims that extracranial–intracranial arterial bypass is good for ischemic brains? (The EC/IC Bypass Study Group (1985).

In the year that the paper by Tom Chalmers and his colleagues was published there were only 347 reports of randomized trials. Half a century later, about 50,000 reports of randomized trials were being published every year, with the total number of trial reports by then exceeding half a million. I am proud to have contributed to this development, to the skepticism that drives it, and to the better informed treatment decisions and choices which have been made possible as a result [99].

The anecdote of how the name "evidence-based medicine" was coined also tells an interesting story. A number of clinicians who demanded that clinical decisions be based on "best" evidence reached critical mass at McMaster University in Hamilton, Ontario, Canada. The group at McMaster, which included Dave Sackett, Gordon Guyatt, Brian Haynes, and Peter Tugwell, began to use the terms "clinical epidemiology" [100,101] and "critical appraisal" to describe their new approach to medicine. In 1990, Gordon Guyatt assumed the position of Residency Director of the Internal Medicine Program at McMaster, where he was charged with several tasks including justifying the innovative approach to medicine and advertising to prospective medical students. In the spring of 1990, Guyatt presented plans for changing the curriculum to the members of the Department of Medicine, many of whom were unsympathetic. Guyatt initially suggested describing the new approach as "scientific medicine." Those already hostile apparently became incensed at the implication that they had previously been "unscientific." Guyatt's second try at a name for McMaster's philosophy, "evidence-based medicine," turned out to be a catchy one. The term initially appeared in an information document aimed at prospective or new students in the autumn of 1990. The relevant passage was:

> Residents are taught to develop an attitude of "enlightened scepticism" towards the application of diagnostic, therapeutic, and prognostic technologies in their day-to-day management of patients. This approach, which has been called "evidence-based medicine". . . The goal is to be aware of the evidence on which one's practice is based, the soundness of the evidence, and the strength of inference the evidence permits. The strategy employed requires a clear delineation of the relevant question(s); a thorough search of the literature relating to the questions; a critical appraisal of the evidence, and its applicability to the clinical situation; a balanced application of the conclusions to the clinical problem [102].

2.3 Original definition of EBM

EBM was initially defined as follows:

> Evidence-based medicine de-emphasizes intuition, unsystematic clinical experience, and pathophysiological rationale as sufficient grounds for clinical decision making and stresses the examination of evidence from clinical research [12].

The terms "clinical experience," "pathophysiologic rationale" and "clinical research" require some clarification here – much more will be said in upcoming chapters.

By "clinical experience" EBM proponents mean expert opinion that is *not* based explicitly on available empirical evidence. While this may be surprising, pre-EBM "methods" often failed to require that existing evidence be considered when making recommendations about the effects of medical therapies. A National Institutes of Health (NIH) report in 1990 in the USA, for example, praised the "expert consensus" method:

> Group judgment methods are perhaps the most widely used means of assessment of medical technologies in many countries. The consensus development conference is a relatively inexpensive and rapid mechanism for the consideration and evaluation of different attributes of a medical technology including, for example, safety, efficacy, and efficiency, among many others [103].

Besides the USA, official representatives from Canada [104], Denmark [105], Finland [106], the Netherlands [107], Norway [108], Sweden [109], and the UK [110] supported the report.

To be sure, the experts on the consensus panel were supposed to review the available evidence. However, the connection between the consensus statement and the best available evidence was often spurious. For example, Antman *et al.* [111] found that even textbook recommendations (written by experts) for treatments intended for heart attack routinely

> . . . failed to mention important advances or exhibited delays in recommending effective preventive measures. In some cases, treatments that have no effect on mortality or are potentially harmful continued to be recommended by several clinical experts.

By "pathophysiologic rationale" ("mechanistic reasoning") EBM proponents mean inferences from (supposed) facts about the underlying pathological and physiological mechanisms of health and disease to conclusions that a treatment will or will not have effects. For example, the belief that antiarrhythmic drugs would reduce mortality was based on (supposed) facts about the causes of mortality (arrhythmias) and the mechanism of action of antiarrhythmic drugs.

Unlike mechanistic reasoning, "clinical research" (I will use the term "comparative clinical study") does not rely directly on *how* the intervention might produce an outcome, and instead involves directly observing the putative outcome relative to the putative outcome produced by a control treatment. A famous example of a comparative clinical study is the Cardiac

Arrhythmia Suppression Trial (CAST), which began in 1987. The trial was designed to test whether antiarrhythmic drugs would reduce mortality in patients who had suffered from myocardial infarction (heart attack). In the study, 27 clinical centres randomized 1455 patients to receive encainide, flecainide, or placebo, while 272 were randomized to receive moricizine or placebo. In April 1989 the encainide, flecainide, placebo arm of the study was discontinued because of excess mortality in the experimental groups; 33 of 730 patients (4.5%) taking either encainide or flecainide had died after an average of 10 months follow-up, while only 9 of 725 patients (1.2%) taking placebo had died from arrhythmia and non-fatal cardiac arrest over the same time period [112]. The experimental drugs also accounted for higher total mortality (56 of 730, or 7.7% in the treatment group versus 22 of 725 or 3.0% in the "placebo" group). Similar negative results were soon found for moricizine [113].

However, EBM proponents do not view all comparative clinical studies as equal: randomized trials are deemed to provide the best evidence for therapeutic effects [12]. As the source for the view that randomized trials provide better evidence, the authors of that 1992 paper cite a 1981 article in the *Canadian Medical Association Journal*: "How to read clinical journals: V: To distinguish useful from useless or even harmful therapy." The article includes careful instructions for helping clinicians decide whether a journal article is worth reading. If the reader's intent is "to distinguish useful from useless or even harmful therapy," then they should "discard at once all articles on therapy that are not about randomized trials" [114].

Another central aspect of the EBM system of evidence that is not explicit in the definitions is the belief that *all* the relevant evidence must be considered before making a decision. The 1992 paper implicitly supports the use of "systematic reviews" (synthesis of all the relevant evidence) when they describe positive ways in which the new paradigm has manifested itself:

> Textbooks that provide a rigorous review of available evidence, including a methods section describing both the methodological criteria used to systematically evaluate the validity of the clinical evidence and the quantitative techniques used for summarizing the evidence [12].

The rationale for the view that all relevant evidence must be considered is self-evident and supported by what philosophers call the "principle of total evidence" [115]. If there were 100 trials, 99 of which gave a "negative" result (where, say, the new drug appeared to be harmful), while 1 had a "positive" result (where the drug appeared helpful), it would obviously

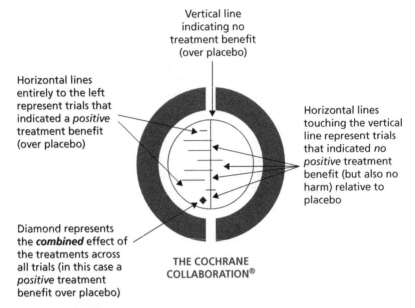

Figure 2.1 The Cochrane Collaboration Logo.

be a mistake to take the single positive trial as definitive and ignore the remaining 99 studies.

The Cochrane Collaboration Logo (Figure 2.1) reveals pictorially the serious problem with failing to consider all the relevant evidence. The horizontal lines in the logo in Figure 2.1 represent a series of trials that tested the benefits of a short inexpensive course of corticosteroids for women about to give birth prematurely. The outcome of interest was infant mortality due to complications of immaturity. In the figure, horizontal lines touching the vertical line indicate that there is no clear benefit of the drug. If the entire horizontal line lies to the left of the vertical line, it indicates that the drug had a positive benefit in that trial. A smaller horizontal line indicates that the result is more precise. The diamond represents the combined effect of the treatment in all the studies.

The first trial was conducted in 1972, and did not find a positive benefit for the drug. Many further smaller trials were conducted over the next two decades, and they were inconsistent. Some found a mild benefit, while others found no benefit. Had systematic reviews been conducted before each new study, however, the positive benefit of the drug would have been conclusively demonstrated as early as 1981.

Not only were all the trials conducted after 1981 a waste of scarce resources, but the uncertainty as to the effects of the drug led to thousands of unnecessary deaths between 1981 and 1995.

What made the case more striking is that Patricia Crowley *did* conduct a systematic review that revealed the effectiveness of the steroid therapy in 1981 [116]. The review found four studies of sufficiently high quality [117–120]. Combined, there were about 1000 babies who received antenatal steroids and a similar number who received placebo. Of those who received antenatal steroids, 70 died, while 130 in the placebo group died. The difference was statistically significant, and clinically relevant. Crowley updated her review over the next few years, uncovering other trials that had been conducted between 1972 and 1979, as well as several that had been conducted afterwards. She published an updated review in 1989 [121].

The NIH, apparently ignorant of the Crowley review, began recruiting for a large-scale trial in 1984. It is unlikely, however, that any parents would have agreed to enter a randomized trial (and risk getting a placebo) after 1981 had they known about Crowley's original review. Unfortunately, the rate of antenatal steroid use for women who were about to give birth prematurely rarely rose above 20% until 1995 when the results of the investigation were published [122]. The failure to consider all the relevant evidence is therefore a tragic travesty of the duty to conduct ethical research.

Another excellent reason to conduct systematic reviews is their ability to detect small but important effects. Many individual trials are too small to detect these modest effects. However, when the effect is important (as it was in the Cochrane Logo example), small effects can obviously be highly relevant. The problem with an insufficient number of participants can be solved either by conducting a much larger study or by combining the results of all the smaller studies in a systematic review.

Another benefit of systematic reviews is that it avoids conducting research if the answer to the research question is already known. In order to learn whether the question has been answered, we must obviously systematically search the literature.

The particular methods for conducting systematic reviews are of course subject to legitimate criticism [43]. However, I will for the most part set aside the practical problems with systematic reviews and take it as given that systematic reviews are methodological necessities for *all* evidence, whether from randomized trials, observational studies, mechanistic reasoning, or even expert judgment. We are still left, of course, with the question of what types of studies we should conduct systematic reviews of.

To sum up, EBM proponents initially took comparative clinical studies, preferably randomized trials, as providing stronger evidence than mechanistic reasoning and expert opinion or judgment. Indeed most early EBM "hierarchies" of evidence did not allow *any* role for mechanistic reasoning, and placed expert judgment below uncontrolled observations [22,23,123].

Armed with the new rules of evidence, EBM practitioners unearthed dozens of examples where comparative clinical studies revealed that treatments adopted based on mechanistic reasoning or lower-quality comparative clinical studies were harmful (even fatal) or useless (see Chapters 5, 10 and 11) [124]. Similarly Iain Chalmers has unearthed several examples where failure to conduct systematic reviews has had lethal consequences [125]. If we accept the results from high-quality comparative clinical studies as definitive, then it appears as though EBM has saved countless lives.

In spite of appearing to support a methodology that saves lives, EBM proponents were wary that they were challenging the status quo (i.e. deferring to authoritative experts and taking mechanistic reasoning as sufficient) and that they would come under attack.

2.4 Reaction to criticism of the EBM system of evidence: more subtle, more or less the same

Early proponents denied that EBM ignored clinical experience and intuition, and mechanistic reasoning. In a subsection of the 1992 paper entitled "Misapprehensions about evidence-based medicine," proponents considered and answered the potential objections as follows.

Misinterpretation 1: EBM ignores clinical experience and clinical intuition.

Correction: On the contrary, it is important to expose learners to exceptional clinicians who have a gift for intuitive diagnosis, a talent for precise observation, and excellent judgment in making difficult management decisions. Untested signs and symptoms should not be rejected out of hand. They may prove extremely useful and ultimately be proved valid through rigorous testing. The more the experienced clinicians can dissect the process they use in diagnosis, and present it clearly to learners, the greater the benefit. Similarly, the gain for students will be greatest when clues to optimal diagnosis and treatment are culled from the barrage of clinical information in a systematic and reproducible fashion.

Misinterpretation 2: Understanding of basic investigation and pathophysiology plays no part in EBM.

Correction: The dearth of adequate evidence demands that clinical problem-solving must rely on an understanding of underlying pathophysiology (when there are no comparative clinical studies). Moreover, a good understanding of pathophysiology is necessary for interpreting clinical observations and for appropriate interpretation of evidence (especially in deciding its generalizability).

While these corrections clarify the importance of expertise and mechanistic reasoning in EBM, they do not go so far as to allow any evidential role for expertise or mechanistic reasoning. Experts are important role models, teachers, and intuitive diagnostic agents, but not for providing evidence that a therapy works. Likewise, EBM proponents claimed that mechanistic reasoning was required when there is no better evidence, and for generalizing the results of comparative clinical studies, but not for making general claims about the effects of medical therapies (see Chapter 10).

In later definitions, EBM proponents make more explicit reference to mechanistic reasoning and expert judgment. For example, in the first (1997) edition of the textbook *Evidence-based Medicine: How to Practice and Teach EBM*, and in a letter to the *British Medical Journal*, Dave Sackett and others defined EBM as follows:

> Evidence based medicine is the conscientious, explicit, and judicious use of current best evidence in making decisions about the care of individual patients. The practice of evidence based medicine means integrating individual clinical expertise with the best available external clinical evidence from systematic research. By individual clinical expertise we mean the proficiency and judgment that individual clinicians acquire through clinical experience and clinical practice. . . . By best available external clinical evidence we mean clinically relevant research, often from the basic sciences of medicine, but especially from patient centred clinical research into the accuracy and precision of diagnostic tests (including the clinical examination), the power of prognostic markers, and the efficacy and safety of therapeutic, rehabilitative, and preventive regimens [32,92].

The authors of the second definition of EBM appear superficially to have made concessions to the roles of clinical expertise and evidence from the "basic sciences." However, it is quite clear that their view about the strength of evidence, expressed in the hierarchy described earlier, did not shift. Clinical expertise, for example, is important for *practicing* EBM, but they do not allow any role for expertise (or expert judgment or experience) as evidence that a therapy works.

Similarly, although the newer definition states that best external evidence "often" comes from the basic science of medicine, they do not allow any role for basic sciences as *evidence* that a therapy works (although they support mechanistic reasoning for other things including generalizing the results of randomized trials).

In fact, if we examine the chapter on appraising evidence, the authors of the first edition of the EBM textbook insist that randomized trials provide the best evidence (unless the effect is so large that more basic observations suffice). Specifically, the textbook contains the following statement: "If you find that the study [of an intervention's effects] was not randomized, we'd suggest that you stop reading it and go on to the next article" [32]. (Again the proviso that randomized trials are the only best evidence for therapy, and even then are not necessary if the effect is dramatic, is also to be found in the same text on page 94.) One can only conclude that the authors of the text are merely paying lip service to the importance of mechanistic reasoning as evidence that a therapy has its putative effects.

In short, while the definition on the first pages of the EBM text appears to contradict the hierarchy of evidence presented earlier, in fact the EBM position on *evidence* (at least evidence for therapeutic effects) remains unchanged: comparative clinical studies, preferably from randomized trials, are deemed to provide better evidence than mechanistic reasoning and clinical expertise.

The second (2000) edition of the EBM textbook appeared to make even more concessions to clinical expertise and mechanistic reasoning. The authors of the second edition define EBM as follows:

> Evidence-based medicine (EBM) is the integration of best research evidence with clinical expertise and patient values.
>
> By *best research evidence* we mean clinically relevant research, often from the basic sciences of medicine ["mechanistic reasoning"], but especially from patient-centered clinical research into the accuracy and precision of diagnostic tests (including the clinical examination), the power of prognostic markers, and the efficacy and safety of therapeutic, rehabilitative, and preventive regimens. New evidence from clinical research both invalidates previously accepted diagnostic tests and treatments and replace them with new ones that are more powerful, more accurate, more efficacious, and safer.
>
> By *clinical expertise* we mean the ability to use our clinical skills and past experience to rapidly identify each patient's unique health state and diagnosis, their individual risks and benefits of potential interventions, and their personal values and expectations.
>
> By *patient values* we mean the unique preferences, concerns and expectations each patient brings to a clinical encounter and which must be integrated into clinical decisions if they are to serve the patient [33].

The most recent (2005) edition of the EBM textbook offers a slight modification to the 2001 definition. In addition to patient values, they note that "patient circumstances" are important. By patient circumstances they mean "their individual clinical state and the clinical setting" [34]. Yet once again, when it comes to appraising evidence, randomized trials remain at the pinnacle of a hierarchy [33,34], while expertise and mechanistic reasoning are omitted altogether [19,126] or are at the very bottom [20,21].

To summarize this chapter, the EBM position on evidence, namely that (systematic reviews of) comparative clinical studies, preferably randomized trials, provide better evidence than mechanistic reasoning and expert judgment has remained more or less unchanged. EBM has, however, emphasized the importance of expertise in several other roles, including intuitive diagnosis, teaching, and role modeling (see Chapter 11).

CHAPTER 3

What is good evidence for a clinical decision?

And yet, I am quite ready to admit that there is a method which might be described as "the one method of philosophy". But it is not characteristic of philosophy alone; it is, rather the one method of all rational discussion, and therefore of the natural sciences as of philosophy. The method I have in mind is that of stating one's problem clearly and of examining its various proposed solutions critically.

—KARL POPPER [3]

3.1 Introduction

This book is an evaluation of the EBM view of what counts as "good" evidence. The strength of evidence depends on what the evidence is *for*. Given that EBM was initially designed to help clinicians make decisions in routine practice [11,32], "good" evidence should be evidence that is useful for making clinical decisions. To be sure, decisions about whether to use an intervention depends on many non-evidential variables, including patient values and cost. But there are several, often overlooked potential features of evidence itself that can, and should, be considered valuable when assessing the strength of evidence. I will argue that good evidence for clinical decisions should be "clinically effective" which means that the treatment has (1) patient-relevant benefits that outweigh any harms, (2) is applicable to the patient being treated, and (3) is the best available option.

The Philosophy of Evidence-Based Medicine, First Edition. Jeremy Howick.
© 2011 Jeremy Howick. Published 2011 by Blackwell Publishing Ltd.

3.2 Evidence *for* clinical effectiveness

Strong evidence that a treatment has "effects" is, by itself, unhelpful. I have indubitable experiential evidence that typing on a computer has an effect on my fingers but such an effect is rarely relevant in clinical practice. Likewise, evidence that a chemical in a drug binds to a cell receptor in a rat may well be the first step in a very fruitful research programme, but it does not, by itself, matter to a doctor or a patient in routine practice. In other cases irrelevance to doctors and patients in routine practice is more difficult to spot. Imagine a pharmaceutical representative enters a doctor's office with evidence that a new drug is highly effective in lowering cholesterol. The doctor, who has been trained in EBM, critically appraises the trial and finds it sound. The trial employed concealed random allocation, as much blinding as feasible, and intention-to-treat analysis. In short, the doctor has good reason to believe that the drug does indeed reduce cholesterol. However, the doctor points out four reasons why she cannot yet accept that the evidence is sufficient for supporting the decision to use the drug in routine practice.

3.2.1 To be useful in clinical practice, the outcomes must be patient-relevant

Lowering cholesterol is not, by itself, a patient-relevant outcome. Patient-relevant outcomes are, in brief, those that make people live better or longer. The notion of living "better" is philosophically charged [127–133], and it is beyond the scope of this work to consider this issue in any detail. At the same time, it is quite clear that some outcomes do improve length or quality of life far more than others. Reducing pain or debilitating fatigue, for example, is far more likely to be relevant to a patient than reducing cholesterol (although reducing cholesterol may predict patient-relevant outcomes).

Many EBM proponents refer to evidence for patient-relevant outcomes as "patient-oriented evidence that matters" (POEMs) [134–136]. Many outcomes, including reducing arrhythmias and lowering cholesterol, are *surrogates* for patient-relevant outcomes such as reduced mortality or morbidity. Unfortunately, as we shall see in Chapter 8 (on "mechanistic reasoning"), links between surrogate and patient-relevant outcomes are rarely well established.

3.2.2 To be useful in clinical practice, the benefits must outweigh the harms

An intervention might have positive effects on patient-relevant outcomes, but negative side-effects that outweigh any positive benefit. For example, beta-blockers are effective for treating hypertension, but they are also effective for hampering male sexual functioning [137]. Or the Halsted radical mastectomy, used for almost 100 years beginning in the late 1890s, reduced *local* recurrence of breast cancer (surgeons did not leave much local flesh in which the cancer could recur) but had no effect on overall mortality from cancer, and had "side-effects" of surgical complications (including death) and of terribly disfiguring women [138,139]. Likewise, antiarrhythmic drugs reduce heart arrhythmias but increase mortality. We would not generally want to call an intervention whose negative side-effects outweighed its positive benefits "effective." Ashcroft [137] puts this point succinctly:

> From a prescriber's point of view, and from a consumer's, it would be a misuse of language to say that a drug whose side-effects are such that they outweigh its benefits is effective.

In order to calculate whether the benefits outweigh the harms, we require an estimate of the effect size. It is not enough for a treatment to simply have *some* benefit – the benefit must be large enough to counteract the harms. Unfortunately, the way many trial results are presented (in terms of "statistical significance" or "relative risk reduction"[1]) can be misleading and do not allow us to make a cost–benefit analysis. In Worrall's words:

> Suppose, unrealistically but for sake of a particularly telling example, only 1 in a million of those whom medics propose to treat with some prophylactic medicine will on average develop some outcome (say stroke within the next 5 years) if left untreated. Then if that medicine reduces the average rate to 0 then this will of course represent a 100% relative risk reduction [140].

Several well-known trials reveal quite small absolute effects. For example, consider the Prevention of Cardiovascular Events and Death with Pravastatin in Patients with Coronary Heart Disease and a Broad Range of Initial Cholesterol Levels, authored by the Long-term Intervention with Pravastatin

---

[1]If we call the event rate (say, the number of strokes) in the experimental group the EER, and the event rate in the control group the CER, the absolute risk reduction (ARR) is simply EER − CER. The relative risk reduction (RRR) is then (EER − CER)/CER. In the example Worrall cites, the EER is 1/1 000 000 and the CER is 0. Therefore, the ARR is 1/1 000 000 and the RRR is 1.

in Ischaemic Disease (LIPID) Study Group. The authors of the LIPID study report a 22% relative reduction in risk of mortality, whereas the *absolute* risk reduction for mortality was 1.9% [141]. While the authors reported no "significant" adverse effects, Worrall is correct to point out that the very act of taking medication can be viewed as a harmful side-effect [140]. Moreover, adverse events are often under-reported (see Chapter 12). Because of the confusion caused by reporting outcomes in terms of relative risk reduction, EBM proponents advocate a measure of effect size directly related to the absolute effect size (the inverse) they call the "number needed to treat" (NNT), which tells us how many people we would need to treat in order to achieve one positive outcome. In the imaginary example Worrall cites above, the NNT would be 1 million. Meanwhile, the 1.9% absolute effect of pravastatin cited in the LIPID study would lead to an NNT of 53. While these small effects may be important – in the LIPID study they certainly were – the point here is that in order to determine whether the benefits outweigh the harms we require a measure of absolute effect size such as the NNT. Similar tiny effects that are misleadingly reported using relative risk reductions include the CARE [142] and GISSI-3 [143] studies (see Worrall [140] for useful discussion).

3.2.3 To be useful, the results of a study must apply to patients in routine practice – the study must have "external validity"

Third, claims that a treatment has effects – even where those effects are patient relevant and where the benefits outweigh the harms – are relativized to a particular group. An intervention might have a patient-relevant benefit for one group but fail to have those effects for another. For example even the most effective antidepressants for adults are not effective for children [144,145]. In another example, the drug benoxaprofen (Oraflex in the USA and Opren in Europe) proved effective in trials for 18–65 year olds, but killed a significant number of elderly patients when it was introduced in routine practice [47]. The problem with applying study results to individual patients in routine practice, often referred to as the problem of "external validity," is exacerbated by the fact that up to 90% of potentially eligible participants for a trial are excluded according to often poorly reported and even haphazard criteria [43,146–148], and only a fraction of the target population are potentially eligible for trials [149]. For a comprehensive treatment of the very real problem with applying study results to individuals see the papers by Rothwell and colleagues [150–152]. In this book, especially in Chapters 5 and 11, I will argue that potential problems with external validity notwithstanding, the EBM methodology remains the one that is *most likely* to tell us what will help individual patients.

Before our doctor accepts the trial of cholesterol-lowering agents (even if they did have overwhelmingly positive patient-relevant benefits) as effective for her patients, she must know that her patients are sufficiently similar to those in the trial.

Recent evidence-ranking systems have partly recognized the importance of clinical relevance when they increase the "quality" of evidence for including patient-centered outcomes, and when the results apply "directly" to the target population [19].

However, more work needs to be done before our doctor accepts evidence as good for *use*. This brings us to our fourth and final feature of "clinical effectiveness" it should include information about available alternatives.

3.2.4 To be useful for clinical practice, the treatment must be the best available option

A trial might demonstrate beyond any reasonable doubt that our cholesterol-lowering agent is *clinically effective*, but unless it compares the intervention's effects with other therapies, the evidence is not useful for clinical decision-making. We saw above, for example, that typical cholesterol-lowering drugs demonstrate less than a 2% absolute risk reduction in mortality over "placebos." In lay terms, it means that 50 people have to take cholesterol-lowering agents in order to prevent one death. The point here is not that cholesterol-lowering agents have small absolute effects, but rather that before a doctor accepts evidence that a new drug is clinically effective as evidence *for use*, she must know (among other things) what the relative benefits and harms of the competing treatment are. There are several other potentially effective strategies for reducing heart disease, including other cholesterol-lowering agents, exercise [153–156], diet [157], and meditation. Before a doctor or patient chooses a cholesterol-lowering drug, they should be aware of the benefits and risks of the available alternatives. All too often, however, new agents are compared with "placebo" and comparative information about other therapies is left to hand-waving.

The NIH in the USA have recently recognized the importance of comparing the effects of alternative treatments and intends to spend $400 million on comparative effectiveness research (CER) [158,159]. At the same time, the importance of CER has not yet filtered through to most evidence-ranking systems. However, the "hierarchy" from the new Oxford Centre for Evidence-Based Medicine (CEBM) contains a warning that the relative effects of available alternatives should be considered before making a clinical decision [160].

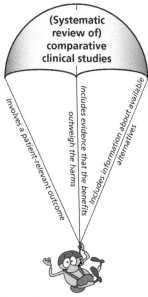

Hypothesis that a treatment is
clinically effective

Figure 3.1 Pictorial representation of what (should) count as "high-quality" evidence for *clinical* effectiveness.

3.3 Strong evidence tells us what?

In order to assess the strength of evidence, we need to know what the evidence is *for*. Given that EBM was designed to help clinical decisions, "good" evidence for clinical decisions has three essential features (Figure 3.1):

1 it tells us whether an intervention's positive patient-relevant benefits outweigh its harms;
2 it applies to individuals in routine practice; and
3 it includes information about available alternative interventions.

The latest EBM evidence-ranking system takes some, but not all, of these elements into account when rating the quality of evidence. The authors of the Grading of Recommendations Assessment, Development and Evaluation (GRADE) system [19] employ a three-step process (Figure 3.2) to decide whether a treatment's putative effects are strongly supported by evidence. First, they assign a "high" grade to randomized trials or a "low" grade to observational studies. Second, observational studies can be "upgraded"

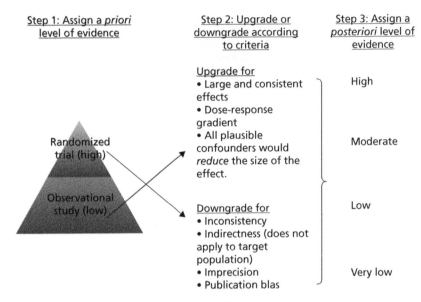

Figure 3.2 The GRADE system for ranking evidence.

for (among other things) demonstrating large effects, and randomized trials can be downgraded for (among other reasons) whether the results are likely to apply to individuals in routine practice. Third, observational studies or randomized trials get assigned "high," "moderate," "low" or "very low." In addition to considering whether the results are likely to apply to patients in routine practice, the results of this chapter suggest that the GRADE system should allow evidence to be upgraded if (i) the study provides evidence that the benefits outweigh the harms, and (ii) whether the study provides evidence of the relative effects of other available interventions.

PART II

Do randomization, double masking, and placebo controls rule out more confounding factors than their alternatives?

CHAPTER 4

Ruling out plausible rival hypotheses and confounding factors: a method

…when you have eliminated the impossible, whatever remains, however improbable, must be the truth.

—Sir Arthur Conan Doyle [161]

The emphasis of EBM on scepticism and uncertainty – we will never be sure about the magnitude of the effects of our treatments or the power of our diagnostic tests – is central to the [EBM] approach and agrees with the philosophical view that scientific knowledge is never complete and ultimately fallible.

—B. Djulbegovic, G.H. Guyatt & R.E. Ashcroft [4]

Over the last millennia, philosophers have proposed many solutions to the problem of how we can justify claims that we know anything. No single attempt has gained widespread agreement, and I will not attempt to solve the problem here. Instead, I will argue for the view that good evidence rules out plausible rival hypotheses. This commonsensical view is embodied in the question Bradford Hill demands we ask before accepting a hypothesis: "Is there any other way of explaining the set of facts before us? Is there any other answer which is more likely than cause and effect?" [2].

I take the "scientific common sense" intuition to be uncontroversial: if there is a rival that remains highly plausible in light of the evidence, then, *ceteris paribus*, it would be irrational to take the evidence as support for the experimental hypothesis. The following real example illustrates the problem with rival hypotheses. In 1968 Woodruff and Dickinson reported that dexamethasone (a steroid) "had a dramatic, and probably life-saving effect" on a man who had been comatose due to malaria for 24 hours. It could be, of course, that in the single case Woodfuff and Dickinson described the dexamethasone *did* cause the dramatic recovery. But patients sometimes recover spontaneously from malarial comas. To learn whether dexamethasone was responsible for the cure in this case we would require access to the "counterfactual" situation where the same person in the same condition at the same time did not receive dexamethasone. This is clearly impossible.

As a surrogate for the impossible, researchers give the experimental treatment (such as dexamethasone) to some people (the "experimental" or "test" group) and compare the outcomes for them with those of another group who do not receive the experimental treatment (the "control" group). Sometimes there is more than one experimental group and more than one control group, but I will restrict myself unless otherwise stated to the simple case with one experimental group and one control group. For example, in a real trial of dexamethasone versus "placebo," the drug appeared to prolong the coma [162].

A problem with this surrogate solution, however, is that there are an indefinite number of differences between any two groups that could conceivably account for recovery from a coma that have nothing whatsoever to do with the experimental drug. For example, the group taking dexamethasone could have been younger, healthier, come from a different socioeconomic class, or taken more exercise, and these factors could affect recovery from malaria. No two peoples' or groups' age, hair length, amount of exercise, health, amount of meat consumed are exactly the same. While many of these differences might appear trivial or irrelevant (more on this below), it is difficult to specify in advance which factors are important. Moreover, there are an indefinite number of them, so we cannot specify a list that we can guarantee to be complete, so even if their effects were trivial they could produce a significant combined effect. Differences between groups at the outset of a study are known as "baseline differences" and a trial that has baseline differences is often claimed to have suffered from *selection bias*.

Things get more challenging when we consider what happens after patients are allocated to the experimental or control groups. If people believe they are receiving the latest and "best" experimental treatment, then quite independently of whether the treatment is effective, their beliefs *could* produce positive outcomes (or, in the case where the trial has "subjective outcomes," cause the patient to *report* a better outcome). Contrariwise, if people believe they are not getting the experimental treatment, then their negative expectations could have negative effects (or negatively affect how they report their outcomes). In our example, if the people receiving dexamethasone knew they were getting the "real" treatment, and the people receiving a "placebo" knew they were receiving a "mere" placebo, then the expectations regarding recovery might be different, and this could influence how much more quickly those taking "real" dexamethasone recover (or report recovery).

Similarly, if the caregivers knew which people received the test treatment, they might lavish more attention on them. Or, believing that those taking the test treatment do not require special attention, might spend more of their scarce time with the patients in the control group. This differential behavior could affect the outcome.

Differing participant expectations and dispenser attitudes are often collectively referred to as types of *performance bias*. Differences between groups "at baseline" (causing selection bias) and differences that arise as a result of patients and dispensers knowing who is receiving the experimental treatment (causing performance bias) present *alternative explanations* for any apparent benefit of a treatment.

More generally, relevant differences between experimental and control groups are referred to as *confounders* or *confounding factors*. EBM proponents claim that randomized trials provide better evidence than observational studies because the former allegedly rule out more confounding factors. With that in mind, it is worthwhile considering the definition of "confounding factor" in some detail. A confounding factor has the following three properties [34].

1 *The factor potentially affects the outcome.* More people in the experimental arm of the trial might have red hair, but since red hair is unlikely to affect most outcomes, on the basis of current knowledge (which is invariably incomplete; see below), it does not satisfy the first condition for being a confounder. Indeed Diana Elbourne and Joanna Harding tested the hypothesis that red-headed women bled more heavily after giving birth and found that it did not [163,164]. On the other hand, age is more likely to affect how quickly people recover from colds, so age satisfies the first condition for being a confounder.

2 *The factor is unequally distributed between experimental and control groups.* If the average age in the experimental group is sufficiently similar to that in the control group, then age does not satisfy the second condition for being considered a confounder.

3 *The factor is unrelated to the experimental intervention.* Ascorbic acid (the "active" ingredient in vitamin C tablets) is both potentially a determinant of the outcome and unequally distributed between groups, but would not be a confounder in a trial of the effects of vitamin C because

it is related to the experimental intervention (it *is* the characteristic feature of the experimental intervention), so it does not satisfy the third condition for being considered a confounder.

Each confounding factor provides a potential alternative explanation for the results of a clinical trial.

However, a problem immediately arises with the first condition: there is an indefinite number of confounders. Let's say we found that randomized trials rule out certain confounders that observational studies do not. Unless randomized trials ruled out *all* confounders (and they do not; see next chapter), we would still be left with indefinitely more potential confounders that had not been ruled out. An indefinite number minus some definite number is still indefinite. Therefore, both randomized trials and observational studies would be methodologically equivalent in the sense that they both suffered from an indefinite number of potential confounders. Consequently, the method of judging the relative quality of comparative clinical studies according to the extent to which they ruled out confounding does not, by itself, help us distinguish between higher- and lower-quality studies.

The solution to the problem of an indefinite number of confounding factors is that some factors are highly likely to be irrelevant. More people in the experimental group might have red hair, but having red hair is highly unlikely to affect most outcomes [163,164]. Thus, we do not need to consider all potential confounders, but only those that *plausibly* affect the outcome.

To be sure, our intuitions can be mistaken. Having red hair could, in some mysterious way, affect most important outcomes, or be associated with some factor such as social class that more plausibly affects important outcomes. In science and medicine, however, perhaps unlike in classical philosophy [165–167], the class of relevant differences ("plausible" confounders) is more clearly defined, and provided by background knowledge. For instance, background knowledge tells us that placebo effects (including patient expectations and beliefs) are more likely to be confounding when outcomes are "subjective" [168,169]. A subjective outcome involves a patient-reported outcome such as levels of pain, depression, or general well-being. An "objective" outcome, on the other hand, generally involves a third party taking a measurement such as heart rate, blood pressure, hormone levels, measuring chemicals (such as opioids) associated with subjective feelings of pain, or in the most objective outcome of all, noting death. In other cases, however, patient expectations and beliefs are unlikely to affect the outcome and therefore unlikely to be confounders. For example, if we were administering external defibrillation to start a stopped heart (and the patient is unconscious), the patient's expectations and beliefs might not be plausible confounders.

Clinical trials, of course, are not our only source of background knowledge. We have all sorts of information about "mechanisms" of a general kind, both positive and negative: hot, heavily chemical-laden smoke frequently inhaled into the lungs is quite likely to adversely affect the lining; substances diluted to the point that it is likely that not a single molecule of the substance under investigation is left are not likely to have an effect. Moreover, in the case of pain, it is well established that various distractions can affect the perception of pain, quite aside from the distraction of increased expectation of amelioration.

Virtually all philosophers of science have acknowledged the role of background knowledge. Consider the following quotes from Mill and Popper.

> In making chemical experiments, we do not think it necessary to note the position of the planets; because experience has shown, as a very superficial experience is sufficient to show, that in such cases that circumstance is not material to the result [170].

> While discussing a problem we always accept (if only temporarily) all kinds of things as *unproblematic*: they constitute for the time being, and for the discussion of this particular problem, what I call our *background knowledge* [171].

Other philosophers of science who emphasize the importance of background knowledge include Hempel [172], Howson [173], and Worrall [47].

Background knowledge, like the results of clinical trials, is of course fallible. In Popper's words:

> The old scientific ideal of *episteme* – of absolute, demonstrable knowledge – has proved to be an idol. The demand for scientific objectivity makes it inevitable that every scientific statement must remain *tentative for ever*. It may be corroborated, but every corroboration is relative to other statements which, again, are tentative. Only in our subjective experiences of conviction, in our subjective faith, can be "absolutely certain" [3].

Many prominent medical statisticians follow Popper in recognizing that knowledge is fallible. Sir Austin Bradford Hill, for example, states:

> All scientific work is incomplete – whether it be observational or experimental. All scientific work is liable to be upset or modified by

advancing knowledge. That does not confer upon us a freedom to ignore the knowledge we already have, or to postpone the action that it appears to demand at a given time [2].

Meanwhile, Martin Bland asserts that "[n]o piece of research can be perfect and there will always be something which, with hindsight, we would have changed" [174]. Indeed an initial aim of EBM was to emphasize that medical "knowledge" is uncertain [175].

To sum up, "background knowledge" provides us with *tentatively* both a class of rivals that we can assume are plausible. We can therefore judge the quality of a comparative clinical study on how well *plausible* confounders have been successfully ruled out. The reason why ruling out confounders is important is simple: confounding factors provide plausible alternative explanations for any apparent benefit (or lack thereof) of a treatment.

In the remainder of Part 2 I will evaluate whether randomized trials (Chapter 5), double-masked trials (Chapter 6), and placebo-controlled trials (Chapters 7 and 8) rule out more *plausible* confounding factors than other study designs.

CHAPTER 5

Resolving the paradox of effectiveness: when do observational studies offer the same degree of evidential support as randomized trials?

5.1 The paradox of effectiveness

Most EBM "hierarchies" of evidence rank randomized trials *categorically* above observational studies [18,20–23,41]. Yet strict adherence to the EBM view leads to the paradox that what we take to be our most effective therapies, ranging from the Heimlich maneuver to unblock an airway to eating to reverse the effects of starvation, have never been tested in randomized trials. Taking the EBM hierarchy at face value (which, as I will argue below, might be a straw man), it seems to follow that our most effective therapies are not supported by "best" (randomized) evidence. Exploiting this irony, Smith and Pell recommended that EBM proponents volunteer to verify whether parachutes prevent death or major trauma in a randomized trial [30].

No doubt partly motivated by the irony, many have criticized the EBM view that randomized trials offer the best evidence [41,46–48,52,59,64, 140,176,177]. In this chapter I will argue that while most critiques of

The Philosophy of Evidence-Based Medicine, First Edition. Jeremy Howick.
© 2011 Jeremy Howick. Published 2011 by Blackwell Publishing Ltd.

randomized trials are straw men against the EBM position, the EBM view must be modified to overcome the paradox of effectiveness. More specifically, I will contend that categorical hierarchies of evidence placing randomized trials above observational studies can be replaced with the view that comparative clinical studies provide good evidence when the effect size outweighs the combined effect of plausible confounding factors. The most recent EBM hierarchy [19], and other developments in the EBM system [31,178] with a few minor modifications, can be viewed as an operational expression of the view I propose.

To anticipate, I will begin by describing observational studies and randomized trials. While the concept of a randomized trial is rather simple, many philosophers and medical professionals misunderstand its essential features. Randomized trials differ from observational studies in that they are randomized, and that they can (but do not have to) employ double masking and "placebo" controls. Next, I review common critiques of the EBM position. Some, including Howson, Urbach, and Worrall, have argued that randomization does not add (much) methodological benefit. Others, including Cartwright and Mant, note that randomized trials lack external validity. I argue that both critiques are straw men against the EBM view. I conclude that paradox of effectiveness can be overcome by modifying the EBM position on randomized trials.

5.2 Observational studies: definition and problems

The most common observational designs are case studies, case series, case–control studies, cohort studies, and historically controlled studies. A detailed description of all these study designs would take us far afield. Moreover, for the purposes of this chapter it suffices to note the essential features of observational studies that are *not* shared by randomized trials. In controlled observational studies (case studies and case series, while important for identifying new disorders [179], do not involve direct comparisons and I will ignore them here), investigators compare people who take an intervention with those who do not. The investigators neither allocate patients to receive the intervention nor administer the intervention. Instead, they compare records of patients who had taken an intervention and been treated in routine practice with similar patients who had not taken the intervention. The main problems with observational studies are that they suffer from (i) self-selection bias (sometimes called *patient preference bias*), (ii) allocation bias, and (iii) performance bias.

In one typical observational study, Petitti *et al.* [180] compared the records of 2656 women who took hormone (estrogen) replacement therapy (HRT) with 3437 who did not and followed them for 10 or more years to measure rates of coronary heart disease (CHD) and overall mortality. They found that HRT users were only half as likely to die as HRT non-users. In 1991 Stampfer and Colditz [181] conducted a systematic review of all the available observational studies of the effects HRT in preventing CHD (all but one were observational) and confirmed that women taking HRT appeared to be, on average, half as likely to die as women who did not take HRT. They concluded that:

> The preponderance of evidence from the epidemiologic studies strongly supports the view that postmenopausal estrogen therapy can substantially reduce the risk for coronary heart disease...This effect is unlikely to be explained by confounding factors or selection [181].

Based on these observational studies millions of women, including my mother, were prescribed and took HRT to (allegedly) protect against CHD and premature mortality.

However, the observational studies of the effects of HRT, like all observational studies, suffered from the problem that people who choose to take (or are chosen by their doctors to take) HRT are likely to be very different in many ways from people who choose not to take (or are not chosen by their doctors to take) HRT. Those who choose not to take HRT might be older, smoke more, tend to work in more polluted conditions (e.g. in mines), eat fewer vegetables, live in wealthier neighborhoods, or differ in any number of other ways from people who choose to take HRT. These differences are all potential confounders because they could all affect how likely people are to contract CHD or cancer *independent* of whether or not they take HRT. Collectively confounding differences between people in the experimental and control groups at the outset of a study and before the treatment is administered (the "baseline") is often referred to as selection bias. Selection bias arising from the fact that patients choose to take a therapy (they "select" it) is referred to as *self-selection bias.*

To be sure, researchers are well aware of self-selection bias. For example, Petitti *et al.* adjusted for age, smoking, body mass index, alcohol intake, hypertension, marital status, and education, and Stampfer and Colditz were careful to rank the studies in their review according to whether investigators had controlled for age, smoking, and types of menopause. Yet, after considering the effects of these potential confounders, Stampfer and Colditz concluded that the apparent protective effect of HRT is "unlikely to be explained by confounding factors or selection" [181].

Careful adjusting reduces confounding and therefore undoubtedly increases the quality of observational studies. Indeed many high-quality observational studies produce the same results as randomized trials (see below). At the same time, some differences will inevitably prove difficult to adjust for. How, for example, would we control for the possibility that women who chose HRT had richer husbands, ate more vegetables, took public transportation, were more optimistic, or had a more extensive social network? These factors could all subtly influence the risk of CHD but are, to say the least, difficult to measure.

The following example suggests that the mere fact of choosing a treatment can have important effects. In one interesting study researchers found that there was no difference in mortality between men treated with clofibrate and those in the control group (who were treated with "placebo"): the mortality was 20% in both groups. Investigators then found that patients who adhered to the treatment regimen more strictly had a lower mortality (15%) than those who did not adhere strictly (25%) [182]. This study has been replicated with consistent results that have recently been summarized in a systematic review [183]. Together, these studies suggest that something to do with a patient's personality (whether or not they adhere to the treatment regimen) can affect the outcome. Presumably, there are a disproportionate number of adherers among those who chose to take a treatment in an observational study. After all, the choice to take a treatment is to adhere at least at the outset to a treatment regimen. Here we have a confounding difference between the two groups in an observational study – a disproportionate number of adherers in the experimental group – that would be difficult if not impossible to control for in an observational study.

Similar biases arise when caregivers are in charge of deciding whether or not to prescribe a treatment. Caregivers could systematically favor the healthier (or less healthy), richer, or younger patients. They are certainly more likely to prescribe treatments to people who bother showing up for their appointments than those who do not. These differences could also confound the observational study.

Things get worse. Other potentially confounding factors can arise *after* the treatment regimen has begun could further confound any comparison between people who take HRT and those who do not. Once people begin taking HRT, they could receive more attention from their doctors, reinforce their social network, or view themselves as victims and worry more. Potential confounding factors that enter after the intervention (HRT) has been chosen are often referred to as forms of performance bias because they arise during the "performance" phase of the trial during which allocated participants take the treatment.

To summarize, observational studies seem particularly vulnerable to both self-selection bias, allocation bias, and performance bias.

5.3 Randomized trials to the rescue

Randomized trials differ from most observational studies in that they involve random allocation and experimental administration of treatments.

5.3.1 Concealed random allocation and ruling out self-selection bias and allocation bias

Unlike in an observational study where patients choose to take the intervention themselves, participants in a randomized trial are *randomly* allocated to receive either an experimental intervention (such as HRT) or a control. Simple random allocation is a process whereby all participants have the same chance of being assigned to one of the study groups [184]. Restricted randomization involves employing various strategies to ensure that the number of participants, and various characteristics such as sex, are similarly distributed between groups (see Appendix 1). A fair coin toss, random number tables, or (pseudo)-random generators on a computer can achieve this. For example, we might flip a coin and assign the next participant in the queue to receive the experimental intervention if the coin lands "heads" up, and the control if the coin lands "tails" up. In practice, of course, coin tosses are rare. Instead, investigators might have a pile of envelopes that contain randomly generated instructions about which group to assign the next patient.

Randomization, when adhered to, rules out self-selection bias and allocation bias. When a random allocation method is used to allocate people to receive the experimental or control treatment, neither participants nor caregivers can influence who receives the experimental intervention.

However, unless the allocation sequence is *concealed*, randomization can, and is commonly, subverted.

Allocation is particularly easy to decipher (and subvert) when the sequence is "pseudo-random," involving alternation or allocation according to date of birth. Real random allocation sequences are also detectable. For example, investigators have opened envelopes containing the sequence or have held them up to lightbulbs to reveal the assignment sequence. Kenneth Schulz conducted a workshop where investigators anonymously revealed the methods they used to decipher the allocation scheme, and heard many stories similar to the following rather amusing one:

> Still another workshop participant had attempted to decipher a numbered container scheme but had given up after her attempts bore no success. One evening she noticed a light on in the principal investigator's office and dropped in to say hello. Instead of finding the principal investigator, she found an attending physician who also was involved

in the same trial. He unabashedly announced that he was rifling the files for the assignment sequence because he had not been able to decipher it any other way. What materialized almost as curious was her response. She admitted being impressed with his diligence and proceeded to help in rifling the files [185].

Knowledge of the allocation sequence is not dangerous provided that it is not subsequently tampered with. The problem is that once caregivers and participants know what treatment they are allocated to, allocation and self-selection bias become worrisome again. For example, a caregiver who was aware of the allocation sequence might not want the very ill patient to receive the risky experimental intervention and suggest that the patient exercise his or her right to withdraw from the trial, telling the patient to return in a few days to try again, or even reaching for another envelope in the pile until the "right" allocation for that patient is selected. If a caregiver does this systematically, a disproportionate number if ill patients will end up in the control group. As a result, the experimental therapy could appear effective simply because those in the experimental group are healthier. The bias could work in the other direction as well. The clinician might believe that the experimental therapy is the next miracle drug, and make sure that the illest patients are assigned to the experimental group. Violations of the assignment scheme are particularly dangerous when the investigator has a personal or financial interest in the new therapy appearing to be effective.

To avoid tampering with the allocation sequence, concealed allocation is often employed. Concealing allocation involves hiding the knowledge of which group receives the experimental intervention from the investigators and participants. For instance, the envelopes containing the allocation schedule could be marked with the letters A and B instead of "experimental" and "control." Then, whether A refers to the experimental therapy or control therapy could be kept secret. Participants' knowledge of the group to which they are assigned can corrupt the randomization schedule in an analogous way. Participants might have learned about the potential benefits of the new drug from the internet and drop out unless they are assigned to the experimental group. Others might fear potential unknown side-effects of the new drug and drop out unless they are assigned to the control group.

A good early example of concealed random allocation involved the now famous 1948 streptomycin trial.

Determination of whether a patient would be treated by streptomycin and bed-rest (S case) or by bed-rest alone (C case) was made by reference to a statistical series based on random sampling numbers drawn up for each sex at each centre by Professor Bradford Hill; the details of the series were unknown to any of the investigators or to the co-ordinator and were contained in a set of sealed envelopes, each bearing on the outside only the name of the hospital and a number. After acceptance of a patient by the panel, and before admission to the streptomycin centre, the appropriate numbered envelope was opened at the central office; the card inside told if the patient was to be an S or a C case, and this information was then given to the medical officer of the centre [186].

5.3.2 Control

Since all randomized trials are controlled by definition, it is redundant to include the "C" in RCT. Randomized trials all involve comparing the experimental therapy with a control therapy. Although there can, in principle, be more than one test group and more than one control group, I will limit my discussion to the simple case where there is a single experimental and a single control group. The control group can either receive another treatment, a "placebo," or "no treatment." A placebo is a treatment capable of making people believe it is, or could be, the experimental treatment when in fact it is not (more on placebos in Chapters 7 and 8). A sugar pill that is indistinguishable to the senses from vitamin C could be a placebo. "No treatment" controls are difficult to construct in practice. Participants in "no treatment" groups are either basically left alone, in which case the investigators lose control over whether participants choose to treat themselves with some other treatment (perhaps covertly), or they are closely monitored, in which case the effects of being monitored could, indeed has been known to [187,188], have effects.

5.3.3 Trial: the experimental design and ruling out performance bias

A medical study is a trial – an experiment – when the investigators are in control of allocating participants to receive the experimental or control intervention(s), *and* they (or other investigators) are in charge of administering the experimental intervention [174,184,189]. Mill, drawing what might be a more accurate distinction, distinguished "artificial" from "natural" experiments [170]. In observational studies, investigators neither allocate participants to test or control groups nor administer the experimental intervention but rather examine records of patients who have been treated in routine practice.

In theory randomization is not required for experimental allocation. Investigators could allocate people experimentally by alternation, rotation, or date of birth. Such allocation would not be randomized, but since investigators perform the allocation, it would be experimental. A practical advantage of random allocation over other experimental methods for allocation is that it is more difficult to decipher and subsequently subvert.

It is also possible to have random allocation (randomized or not) but not employ experimental administration of the treatment. For example, patients could be randomized to receive the experimental intervention or control, then be treated (or not if the study involved a "no treatment" control) in routine practice. In practice these are called randomized pragmatic trials.

In sum, the experimental nature of randomized trials simply means that investigators allocate to test and control groups and, often, that the treatments are administered experimentally.

Experimental administration of test and control treatments, although not a *necessary* feature of randomized trials, provides randomized trials with two further potential advantageous features over observational studies: randomized trials, but not observational studies, can employ double masking and "placebo" controls.

Briefly (much more to follow in the next chapter), double masking can reduce the potentially confounding influence of several confounding factors that arise from knowledge of who receives the experimental treatment. If patients know they are receiving the latest and best therapy, they might improve because of their beliefs and expectations and not because of the experimental therapy itself. We will see in the next three chapters that people can recover, even quite dramatically, from various ailments simply because they believe they are taking a powerful treatment (or *report* that they are recovering more quickly, which is all that is at issue when the outcome is subjective). For example, depressed patients seem to recover more quickly (or report they recovered more quickly) when they *know* they are receiving a "real" antidepressant drug than they do if they are not sure whether they are taking a "real" antidepressant drug [190–193]. Similarly, investigator attitudes have been known to influence interpretation of rat [195] and human [195] behavior, and also more "objective" measures such as blood cell counts [196]. Besides confounding influences of expectations and beliefs, participant and caregiver knowledge can lead to other confounders including differential drop-out rates and concomitant medication.

To rule out the potentially confounding factors arising from caregiver and participant expectations and beliefs, we can "blind" or "mask" the participants and caregivers in charge of administering the intervention. Masking, like concealment, involves hiding the knowledge of who receives the experimental intervention (see Chapter 5). A "double-blind" or "double-masked" study is a study in which neither the participants who receive the intervention nor caregivers who administer the intervention are aware of who gets the experimental intervention. For example, in a double-blind randomized trial of HRT versus placebo, neither the participants nor the caregivers will know whether the particular pill they take (or administer) is "real" HRT. Not knowing whether they are in the experimental or control group, the participants' expectations, and any effects of these expectations, will not be confounded by the knowledge that they are taking a particular treatment. Similarly, if the physicians who administer the intervention do not know which participants are in the experimental or control groups, their treatment of all participants will not be different because of their knowledge of who is taking the experimental treatment.

Because observational studies involve observations of what happens in routine practice, it is practically impossible for them to be conducted in double-masked conditions. Unless something has gone wrong, caregivers will know what interventions they are administering, and (one hopes) they tell their patients. Exceptions include cases where the healthcare practitioner prescribes something by accident, or if the patient is unconscious.

"Placebo controls" are often required to achieve double masking. In order to deceive trial participants into believing that they *might* be taking the experimental intervention, it must be possible to disguise the control intervention as the experimental intervention. Often the easiest way to achieve this is by designing an intervention that looks superficially like the experimental treatment but which does not have its "characteristic" features. For example, we might design a pill that looks like an HRT tablet but which contains no actual estrogen. Like with double masking, placebo controls are practically impossible to employ in observational studies. In routine practice treatments already have (supposedly) proven effects. To be sure, some treatments prescribed in routine practice are, for all intents and purposes, placebos. For example, doctors will sometimes knowingly prescribe antibiotics for viral infections when the patient demands that something be done, or when the doctor herself would like to appear as though she is doing something. One might argue on this basis that we *could* conduct observational studies with placebo controls. However, this would be practically impossible. For example, not all antibiotics are prescribed for viral infections and without detailed records it would be difficult to identify a control group that had been treated with placebo antibiotics in routine practice.

To summarize this section, the essential feature of a randomized trial is that it involves random allocation to treatment groups. Randomization, provided it were adhered to (which is often impossible unless the allocation is concealed), helps to reduce baseline confounders. The experimental nature of randomized trials permits them to employ two features that are generally unavailable to observational studies designs, namely double masking and placebo controls. These further, potential features of randomized trials allow them to reduce potential performance bias introduced by participant and caregiver knowledge of who receives the experimental intervention.

In spite of its surface appeal, the EBM view that randomized trials belong above observational studies in a hierarchy has been criticized. In the next section I will review the criticisms and argue that they fail, by and large, to undermine the EBM position that randomized trials provide better evidence to observational studies.

5.4 Defending the EBM view that randomized trials provide better evidence than observational studies

In perhaps the most widely cited philosophical critique of the EBM hierarchy, Worrall develops earlier work by Urbach [197] and Howson [49] and adopts an interesting strategy for criticizing the EBM placement of randomized trials at the top of the evidence hierarchy. He considers five potential benefits of randomization, namely:

1 randomization is required for classical hypothesis testing;
2 randomization is required to establish probabilistic causality;
3 randomization controls for all confounders (both known and unknown);
4 randomization controls for allocation bias; and
5 observational studies are "known" to exaggerate treatment effects.

At the end of his analysis he concludes that the only benefit of randomization is that it rules out allocation bias. But because, he argues, this benefit is only modest, well-conducted observational studies often provide equally strong evidence. Along with several other critics, Worrall also argues that observational studies have a greater degree of external validity than randomized trials.

I will set aside the arguments that randomization is required for classical hypothesis testing and to establish probabilistic causes because the EBM method is not directly tied to classical hypothesis testing. In fact EBM has promoted non-classical (Bayesian) methods for diagnostic reasoning. Nor does EBM have a stake in the outcome of the philosophical debate over probabilistic causality (see Appendix 2). Instead I will focus on the arguments that the EBM movement itself can be interpreted to have put forward, namely that randomization controls for all confounders, that randomization controls for allocation bias, and that observational studies are "known" to exaggerate treatment benefits.

To anticipate, I will argue that Worrall's critique of randomized trials is a straw man against the EBM hierarchy of comparative clinical studies. I will then explain why neither observational studies nor other methods solve the problem of external validity. At the same time, more subtle critics are correct to note that the *categorical* position of randomized trials above observational studies in older hierarchies is mistaken: in some, albeit exceptional cases, observational studies can provide equally good evidence.

5.4.1 Worrall's critique of the argument that randomization controls for all known and unknown confounders

EBM proponents (and others) have claimed that randomization controls for all confounders, both known and unknown. The EBM textbook, for example, states:

> Random allocation balances the treatment groups for these and other prognostic factors, even if we don't yet understand the disorder well enough to know what they all are! [32].

To see why this strong claim about the power of randomization is mistaken, imagine we had a trial involving two people, one male and one female. If a fair coin toss decided whether the participants received the experimental intervention, the trial would *necessarily* have serious baseline differences. Either both participants would be in one group, leaving the other empty, or there would be one male (or female) in the control group and one female (or male) in the experimental group. In a real example, a randomized trial compared cognitive group therapy with "no treatment" in 32 patients. The control group had 17 patients (14 female, 3 male) and a total of 44 competing diagnoses (patients could have more than one competing diagnosis),) while the experimental group had 15 patients (11 female, 4 male), 17 with anxiety disorders and a total of 29 with competing diagnoses. These two groups have clear differences (more females, more competing diagnoses in the experimental group, etc.) that are *known* to affect outcomes. For this reason many medical researchers insist that randomization be restricted (see Appendix 1) so that known confounders are distributed equally. For example, Bradford Hill states:

> When the results of a treatment are likely to vary between, say, the sexes or different age groups, then a further extension of this method may be made, to ensure a final equality of the total groups to be compared [2].

Other well-known medical textbooks make similar claims [174,189]. But even if known confounders were equally distributed, it remains possible that *unknown* confounders remain.

It is sometimes claimed, on randomization's behalf, that it controls for unknown confounders as well. The EBM textbook, for example, insists that randomization controls for confounders "even if we don't yet understand the disorder well enough to know what they all are!" [32]. Similar claims are echoed elsewhere:

> [T]he full procedure of randomization [is the method] by which the validity of the test of significance may be guaranteed against corruption by the causes of disturbance which have not been eliminated [by being controlled] [198].
>
> We can equalise only for such features as we can measure or otherwise observe, but we also need unbiased allocation for all other features, some of which we may not even know exist. Only randomisation can give us that, and no form of equalisation can be a satisfactory substitute for it [2].

But if randomization does not guarantee, for example, that males will be equally distributed between groups, then how could randomization distribute some unknown factor equally?

In a *sufficiently large* randomized trial, of course, the law of large numbers will tend to ensure that both known and unknown differences wash out. But most trials are not sufficiently large (see below). However, the argument that randomization does not control for *all* known and unknown confounders is a straw man against the EBM hierarchy for two reasons.

First, statements by EBM proponents that randomized trials control for all known and unknown confounders may have been taken out of context. Three sentences below the quote from the EBM textbook stating that randomization rules out all confounders, the very same text states:

> The reason for insisting on random allocation to treatments is that this comes *closer than any other research* design to creating groups of patients at the start of the trial who are identical in their risk of the events you're trying to prevent [my emphasis] [32].

This is different from claiming that randomization rules out *all* confounding factors.

Just a few pages later, the same textbook suggests that we "double-check to see whether randomization was effective by looking to see whether patients were similar at the start of the trial" [32]. If randomization ruled out all confounders, there would be little need to double-check. While it is important to call mistaken claims about the power of randomization to task, it is unfair to take what EBM proponents have said out of context. Second, even if EBM proponents have not been quoted out of context, they do not require randomization to rule out *all* confounding factors in order to support the view that randomized trials provide superior evidence to observational studies. All they require is for randomized trials to rule out *more* confounding factors than observational studies. Strict random allocation (enforced by concealment) rules out self-selection bias and allocation bias, while non-random allocation methods used in observational studies do not. Then, observational studies cannot (practically) employ double masking or placebo controls to reduce performance bias. While Worrall fails to note that randomized trials rule out patient preference bias and performance bias, he admits that random allocation rules out allocation bias (he calls it "selection bias"), and acknowledges that this is a "cast-iron argument for randomization" [47]. Therefore, according to the rule that the quality of evidence depends on how well it rules out confounding (which Worrall explicitly endorses), all other things being equal (which they may not be – see below) randomized trials provide superior evidence to non-randomized trials (unless observational studies have problems of their own; see below).

5.4.2 Randomized trials exaggerate treatment benefits

The argument that randomized trials rule out more confounders than observational studies is supported by empirical studies suggesting that observational studies provide different (usually larger) effect estimates than randomized trials [199,200]. The comparison is (or should be), of course, between randomized trials and observational studies of similar quality. Quite recently, Lacchetti *et al.* [124] reported 22 cases where observational evidence has been contradicted by subsequent randomized trials. To name a few well-known examples, sodium fluoride appeared to reduce vertebral fractures in an observational study [201] but not in a subsequent randomized trial [202]; vitamin E appeared to reduce major coronary events in a cohort study [203] but not in a large randomized trial [204]; and low-dose aspirin appeared less effective than high-dose aspirin in observational studies [205] but the reverse was true in subsequent randomized trials [206].

In an example I will discuss in some detail, we saw above that HRT appeared to reduce CHD, stroke, and dementia in postmenopausal women in observational studies [181,207]. HRT was also touted, based on observational studies, to reduce the risk of stroke, dementia, and cancer [181,208]. However, subsequent randomized trials suggested that women taking HRT were more likely to get CHD, stroke, dementia, and even breast cancer [209,210] (my mother was among the women who got breast cancer after taking HRT).

Taken alone, however, the fact that randomized trials sometimes produce different results from observational studies does not imply that randomized trials provide the more accurate result [47]. A stubborn supporter of observational studies could insist that the observational studies rather than the randomized trials provided the more accurate effect estimate. Indeed it is viciously circular to assert that randomized trials provide the more accurate result based on any observed differences between the results of randomized trials and observational studies.

However, the vicious circularity can be escaped by appealing to the rule that better evidence rules out more confounding factors. Since, as even Worrall admits, randomized trials rule out allocation bias while observational studies do not, it follows (unless there are other reasons to prefer observational studies) that we should accept randomized trials as superior. In fact (unless we believe that the randomized trials had additional confounders of their own), we should conclude that the observational study provides the wrong result *because* it was likely to have been confounded by allocation bias, self-selection bias, or performance bias.

There are two more objections to the empirical argument that randomized trials provide best evidence. First, several studies suggest that more recent, better-conducted observational studies provide similar effects to randomized trials [36,38]. For instance, Benson and Hartz [36] conclude that there is:

> little evidence that estimates of treatment effects in observational studies reported after 1984 are either consistently larger than or qualitatively different from those obtained in randomized, controlled trials.

Benson and Hartz hypothesize that the reason for the apparent convergence of randomized trial and observational results is that the methodology of observational studies has improved. There would be good reason to celebrate if, in fact, randomized trials and observational studies generally provided sufficiently similar results. After all, randomized trials are sometimes unethical or unfeasible, and can be more expensive to conduct.

Unfortunately, it is far from clear whether observational studies generally provide similar results to randomized trials. Screening for breast cancer, for example, is one of the five issues examined by Concato *et al.* Yet Pocock and Elbourne point out that a more recent meta-analysis of higher-quality randomized trials shows little protective effect of mammography [211]. More generally, as mentioned above, Lacchetti *et al.* have identified 22 cases where randomized trials disagreed with results of observational studies. When the crucial issue is whether observational studies provide evidence as strong as randomized trials, cases where results differ, not where they are the same, are more relevant. Faced with two contradictory studies of similar quality, one randomized and one not randomized, it is rational to bet on the results of the randomized study because the randomized study is less likely to be biased. Indeed anyone who denies this principle should be forced to answer the question "Faced with a high-quality observational study that indicates, say, a benefit of HRT, and a high-quality randomized trial indicating that HRT is harmful, what would you do?"

Similarly, several critics [44,212) raise the more fundamental objection that Concato *et al.* and Benson and Hartz selected an unrepresentative sample of observational studies. They complain, for example, that Concato *et al.* analyze only five therapeutic issues, while Benson and Hartz summarize evidence from 18 therapeutic comparisons in four paragraphs and two figures, which makes their claims difficult to evaluate. Kunz *et al.* [212] assert quite correctly that in order to conclude whether randomized trials routinely provide the same results as randomized trials, "a systematic review that includes all the available evidence…can provide the needed answers." In the absence of such a *systematic* comparison, we cannot conclude that observational studies provide similar results to randomized trials *in general.*

A second objection to the empirical evidence that observational studies produce different (usually larger) effect estimates is that results of randomized trials can also be contradictory. Ioannidis [213] recently analyzed all original clinical research studies published between 1990 and 2003 that had been cited more than 1000 times. Of the 39 randomized trials he identified, 9 (23%) had been contradicted by subsequent studies. In a typical example, a randomized trial of treatments for sepsis suggested that monoclonal antibody to endotoxin could cut mortality in half [214], but a subsequent tenfold larger trial found that the same antibody could *increase* mortality [215]. The main reason for conflicting results of randomized trials appears to be their quality. Many randomized trials are *underpowered* (too small to detect effects) [216], fail to conceal the allocation sequence [217–219], fail to implement double masking [220–222], have effect sizes so small that "statistically significant" results can arise by chance [223–225), and suffer from confounding from other sources [226–229]. Indeed EBM proponents have often lamented the poor quality of research [230–232].

However, it does not follow from the fact that many randomized trials sometimes contradict one another or that randomized trials sometimes suffer from methodological limitations that observational studies are equally reliable. Indeed observational studies seem to contradict one another far more often than randomized trials [213]. Thus, even though randomized trials of differing quality will provide different results, it seems that we are still better off betting on the results of randomized trials than observational studies. At the same time, the inconsistency of randomized trial results confirms the EBM insistence on skepticism and that *all* studies are open to question and do not provide us with absolute truths [4]. In addition, the fact that randomized trials can suffer from methodological limitations suggests that a *categorical* ranking of randomized trials above observational studies might be misleading (see next section).

To recap, randomized trials sometimes contradict the results of observational studies. These empirical studies can be taken as evidence that the biases ruled out by randomization (self-selection bias and allocation bias) have important effects.

5.4.3 Are randomized trials less externally valid than observational studies?

Up to this point, I have considered the arguments that randomized trials rule out more confounding factors than observational studies and concluded that they do. The matter would end here if observational studies did not have any advantages over randomized trials. In fact, many argue that observational studies have a greater degree of external validity than randomized trials [46,47,62,64,140,233]. The problem of external validity is very real, and philosophers have proposed various solutions, including (i) using observational studies, (ii) appealing to mechanistic reasoning [52,56], and (iii) appealing to expert judgment [64]. I will consider the first here, and the other two in Chapters 10 and 11.

Worrall uses the example of benoxaprofen (Oraflex in the USA, Opren in Europe), which proved effective in trials for 18–65 year olds but killed a significant number of elderly patients when it was introduced to routine practice [47]. However, once again this is a straw man against the EBM view that randomized trials provide stronger evidence than observational studies: observational studies suffer from problems of external validity of their own. Worrall's example, for instance, could have arisen from an observational study where the study population differed in some way from the target population. Observational studies, like most randomized trials, only provide average results that are not straightforwardly applicable to individuals unless there was little variation in treatment response. Likewise, it is not generally the case that observational studies use more representative populations than randomized trials. In many cases, of course, randomized trials exclude many participants who would eventually receive the therapy in routine practice [43,146–149]. But this is not a necessary feature of randomized trials. Indeed some randomized trials include almost everyone from the target population. For example, the GISSI-1 trial of thrombolysis for acute myocardial infarction recruited 90% of patients admitted within 12 hours of the event with a definite diagnosis and no contraindications. Meanwhile, not all observational studies have a high degree of external validity [234].

In addition, empirical evidence suggests that *even if* randomized trials appear to involve unrepresentative populations, the results apply to the target population [235–237].

Next, one type of randomized trial, namely *n*-of-1 trials have arguably the highest degree of external validity of any comparative clinical study. In an *n*-of-1 trial, there is only one participant – the patient – and a random allocation method determines whether the participant receives the experimental intervention then the control, or vice versa. For example, a random method might determine whether a participant in an *n*-of-1 study of vitamin C versus placebo might receive the vitamin C for 1 month, then a placebo for the next month, and this process might be repeated several times. Typically such a trial would be conducted in double-masked conditions. If the participant recovered more quickly from colds in the months when taking real vitamin C, we would have evidence that vitamin C was responsible. There would be no issue of the trial results not applying to the individual.

While *n*-of-1 trials are only applicable for relatively stable conditions, there is no real observational equivalent of an *n*-of-1 trial. An observation of one person, for instance, would not be able to distinguish therapeutic effects from natural history or spontaneous remission.

Finally, the problem of external validity is irrelevant unless a study is "internally valid" (in brief, not confounded). With a few exceptions confounded studies provide inaccurate results whose results are unreliable guides to therapeutic effects for those within the trial or to individuals in routine practice.

To summarize this section, the EBM claim that randomized trials in general provide superior evidential support to observational studies stands up to scrutiny. Even critics admit that randomized trials rule out more confounding factors than observational studies. And most critiques of randomized trials apply equally to observational studies. However, this view leaves us with the paradox that our most effective treatments, ranging from the Heimlich maneuver to external defibrillation, appear to be less well supported by evidence than many of our treatments with much smaller effects since their effects have never been tested in randomized trials of any description.

5.5 Overcoming the paradox of effectiveness

The resolution to the paradox of effectiveness involves reconsidering the reason why ruling out confounders is useful: confounders provide an *alternative hypothesis* for the result. For example, it seems that the observational studies of the protective effects of HRT cited above were confounded by differences in the average health of women who chose to take HRT. The differences between women who chose to take HRT and those who did not provided an alternative explanation for the apparent positive result of the study. Instead of HRT "causing" the apparent positive effect, it was likely to have been the better average health of women who actually took HRT.

However, sometimes the confounding factors do *not* provide an alternative explanation for the outcome of a study. For example, selection bias and expectation effects are unlikely to be sufficiently powerful to account for the observed effects of general anesthesia, the Heimlich maneuver, external defibrillation, or parachute use. In these cases, although some plausible confounders have not been ruled out by the design of the study, the large observed effect has swamped the combined effects of any plausible confounders. Thus, the failure to test the effects of these therapies in double-masked placebo-controlled trials should not count against our beliefs, say, that general anesthesia causes reversible loss of consciousness. It remains true in an abstract sense that a less confounded randomized trial would provide a more accurate estimate of the effect size of general anesthesia than an observational study. But as far as evidence that is useful for clinical practice, an observational study whose effect size swamps the combined effect of plausible confounders provides sufficient evidence. Indeed, if a study reveals a dramatic effect, then we might judge that the strength of evidence it provides is greater.

With this in mind, we should change the question we ask when appraising the validity of a study. Rather than simply ask whether it was confounded or where it fits into a categorical hierarchy, we should ask the question "Is the effect size is larger than the combined effect of plausible confounders" [46–48,177,238][2] (Figure 5.1).

Two notes of caution about this more subtle use of evidence are required. First, there are sometimes strong *relative* effects but small absolute effects. Although "weak" causes may be as real as "strong" causes, it takes fewer (or "weaker") confounders to account for a small absolute effect than for a large absolute effect. We therefore must be more careful when inferring from

---

[2]This rule of evidence was inspired by Worrall [46,47] and developed by Howick, Glasziou and Aronson [178]. The remainder of this section is largely borrowed from Howick *et al.* [178].

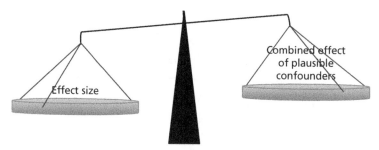

Figure 5.1 The strength of evidence from a comparative clinical study depends on whether the effect size outweighs the combined effect of plausible confounders.

a strong relative (but small absolute) effect that an association is causal. At the same time, in many cases strong relative (but small absolute) effects can provide strong support for the causal hypothesis. For instance, although the increased risk for lung cancer in smokers Bradford Hill cited was extremely low (0.07 per 1000 for non-smokers, 0.57 for smokers), the death rate for lung cancer in cigarette smokers was over nine times the rate for non-smokers and thus provided good evidence for causation.

Second, the effect size must be truly dramatic if we are to be confident in the results of observational studies. Empirical studies reveal that failure to randomize, conceal allocation, and to double mask all exaggerate treatment benefits. While information about the *absolute* size of these effects (see Chapter 3) is not provided, the odds ratios[3] are exaggerated by an average of 41% for failure to conceal allocation, and 17% for failure to double blind. Together, therefore, odds ratios of treatment benefits are likely to be exaggerated by an average of 65% in studies involving unconcealed and unblinded methods.

Appealing to the rule that the effect size should outweigh the combined effect of plausible confounders has several important consequences for the interpretation of comparative clinical studies. First, it allows observational studies to provide equally strong evidence to randomized trials in some cases. Second, it explicitly takes the intuition that effect size should be considered when considering the strength of evidence. A carefully controlled observational study with a large effect could provide stronger evidence than a confounded randomized trial with a small effect. Third, the rule of evidential support I propose suggests that observational studies

---

[3]Odds ratio = (odds of outcome event/odds of no outcome event in control group)/ (odds of outcome event/odds of no outcome event in experimental group).

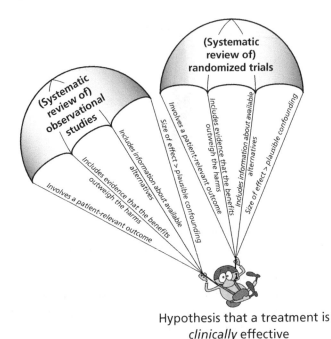

Hypothesis that a treatment is
clinically effective

Figure 5.2 Guidelines for evaluating the strength of evidence from comparative clinical studies. (As always, systematic reviews must be conducted so that all relevant evidence is taken into account.)

could be weighed alongside randomized trials in support of a claim that a treatment produced a clinically relevant benefit (Figure 5.2). Using a hierarchy of evidence encourages researchers to reject observational studies when randomized trials are available. However, if the observational study satisfies the requirement I outline, there is no reason why they should not be weighed together with randomized trials when deciding whether to accept a claim that a medical treatment produced a clinically relevant effect.

The rule of evidence I propose reflects recent developments amongst EBM proponents. For example, Glasziou *et al.* [31] recently argued that under certain conditions (including when effect sizes are dramatic) observational studies provide equally strong evidence to randomized trials. In addition, the latest EBM evidence-ranking system (GRADE; see Chapter 3) allows observational studies to be upgraded for displaying large effects. However, GRADE does not downgrade randomized trials for revealing very small effects. While small effects are often important, it only takes one weak confounding factor to tip the scales and lead to a false positive result. For this reason, my guideline can be more stringent than current EBM standards of evidence.

According to GRADE, randomized trials with a low risk of bias are often ranked "highly." I require that, in addition to being at low risk, the effect size outweigh the combined effects of any residual bias. For example, although most systematic reviews of high-quality randomized trials of selective serotonin reuptake inhibitors (SSRIs) suggest that these drugs enjoy a statistically significant benefit over placebo [239,240], the absolute benefit is modest: a recent study suggests it is 6% (2–9%) [241]. Yet one often overlooked source of confounding in these studies is the identifiable side-effects of the drug. If patients identify the drugs because of the side-effects, then their expectations regarding recovery might be higher than if they knew they were taking a mere placebo. To rule out the possible confounding effect of expectations, "active placebos" that imitate the side-effects of antidepressant drugs need to be employed. A systematic review of antidepressants versus "active" placebos found that the drug less placebo difference was substantially reduced [191]. Besides confounding expectations, systematic reviews of SSRIs (like most systematic reviews) are likely to be confounded to some degree by publication bias [226,242], funding source bias [243], and data mining in the original studies [228]. A careful calculation of the combined effects of these plausible confounders must be made before believing that the benefits of SSRIs over 'placebos' are real. Such calculations have not (to my knowledge) been made, so my proposed rule of evidence, unlike GRADE, does not necessarily support the existence of (non-placebo) effects of SSRIs.

5.6 Conclusion: a more subtle way to distinguish between high- and low-quality comparative clinical studies

Randomized trials rule out the potentially confounding influence of self-selection bias and allocation bias while observational studies do not. Hence, randomized trials will usually provide stronger evidence than observational studies. A common objection to randomized trials is that they do not possess a high degree of external validity. While the problem of external validity is real, it is unclear how observational studies offer a solution. At the same time, strict adherence to early EBM hierarchies leads to the paradox that our most effective therapies, ranging from the Heimlich maneuver to unblock an airway and external defibrillation to start a stopped heart are not supported by "best" evidence. I argued that the paradox can be resolved by replacing categorical hierarchies with the view that comparative clinical studies provide good evidence when the effect size outweighs the combined effect of plausible confounding factors. Figure 3.1 from Chapter 3 can now be amended to take this criterion for appraising comparative clinical studies into account (see Figure 5.2).

Appendix 1: types of restricted randomization

Restricted randomization deviates from simple randomization and comes in several forms. In all cases the purpose of restricted randomization is to equalize known or suspected potential baseline differences. Block randomization, for instance, ensures that the experimental and control groups are in the desired proportion. More specifically, block randomization randomizes n individuals into k treatments of block size m (the sample size must be divisible by the block size). For example, if there were 10 individuals and two study groups, then we might use two blocks, TC and CT, where TC meant "first test treatment, then control" and CT meant "first control, then test treatment." Then, a coin toss would indicate which block (TC or CT), and thus an order, in which the next two participants in the trial would be assigned to study groups [184]. Larger block sizes, and even randomly chosen block sizes, can also be used [174]. Usually, there would be very similar numbers of participants in the test group and in the control group.

Other forms of restriction, including *stratification, weighted randomization*, and *minimization* can be used with or without blocking. The different methods for restricting randomization may be used along with blocking. *Stratified* randomization attempts to keep relevant characteristics, such as age, sex, or disease severity, equal across groups. In a stratified design, participants are organized into various *strata*, and the members of each strata are randomized into the various treatment arms. So, for example, there could be a strata of males. Then this strata would be randomized to the various study groups. With *minimization*:

> the first participant is truly randomly allocated; for each subsequent participant, the treatment allocation is identified which minimizes the imbalance between groups at that time. That allocation may then be used, or a choice may be made at random with a heavy weighting in favor of the intervention that would minimize imbalance (for example, with a probability of 0.8) [244].

Finally, researchers can employ *weighted* randomization. In these cases, the randomization can be weighted so that, on average, more people are assigned to one of the study groups. For further discussion see Bland [174] and Armitage *et al.* [189].

Appendix 2: Worrall's arguments that randomization is required for classical hypothesis testing and establishing probabilistic causes

The logic of classical hypothesis testing

Some medical historians have asserted that classical statistical theory led to the modern randomized trial (the 1948 MRC Streptomycin trial) [245–247]. If, as is sometimes asserted, randomized trials are required for classical hypothesis tests, classical hypothesis tests were useful, then this would be a further advantage of randomization.

However it is unclear whether classical hypothesis testing requires randomization or whether the modern clinical trial requires classical hypothesis testing. Denying that classical hypothesis testing requires randomization, Howson and Urbach [49] state:

> Despite the widespread agreement that significance tests require randomization, expositions of the standard tests that are employed in the analysis of trials, such as the t-test, the chi-squared test, and the Wilcoxon Rank Sum test, barely allude to randomization.

More importantly, the modern clinical trial in particular or the EBM movement in general may not value randomization for statistical reasons. Doll recently stated that randomization was introduced to medical trials in order to reduce allocation bias rather than for any statistical reason. Likewise Chalmers examined the details of the 1948 MRC Streptomycin trial in detail, and found no evidence that Bradford Hill's use of concealed randomization had anything to do with esoteric statistical reasons and more to do with ruling out allocation bias [2,248). Chalmers' finding is supported by Lasagna's 1955 report of the benefits of randomization [249] and at least one other similar investigation [250]. In short, it seems far from obvious that randomization was introduced to conform with classical hypothesis testing. Instead, it seems to have been introduced to medicine for the more commonsensical reason of reducing bias.

There are further reasons to question the link between EBM and classical hypothesis testing: EBM proponents have advocated deviations from classical statistics. To name just a few, EBM proponents have rejected reporting of P-values in favour measures of absolute effect size such as number needed to treat, or NNT, and for emphasizing the importance of non-classical (Bayesian) analysis in diagnostic reasoning. An appendix to the EBM textbook on confidence intervals states "The most appropriate methods [classical or Bayesian] of statistical analysis and presentation must be largely a matter for personal judgment" [34]. In short, even if it is true that classical hypothesis testing requires randomization (which is unclear), EBM proponents have no reason to be, and in fact do not seem to be, necessarily tied to classical statistical analysis. It follows that Worrall's attack of EBM or randomized trials based on their alleged links to classical statistics is a straw man.

Randomization and probabilistic causality

We all accept probabilistic causes. Smoking increases the risk of lung cancer yet not everyone who smokes contracts lung cancer and not everyone who gets lung cancer smokes. Worrall notes that important contributors to the field of probabilistic causality [251–253]

> have explicitly claimed that it follows from their accounts that randomizing in a clinical trial is the vital ingredient in underwriting the claim that there is a *genuinely causal* connection between the treatment and the outcome, rather than a merely associational one (on the assumption, of course, that the outcome of the RCT is positive) [47].

However, it is unclear how randomizing ensures genuine causality by ruling out chance associations or common causes. Imagine, for instance, that we were testing the hypothesis that vitamin C caused speedier recovery from the common cold by randomizing people to get either vitamin C or placebo, and that we found the average recovery time in those who took vitamin C to be much shorter. But of course, being under 40 may also "cause" speedier recovery from the common cold, and simple random allocation may well have resulted in more under-40s in the experimental group. Worrall concludes that the alleged connection between randomization and "genuine" causality is merely the argument that randomization controls for all confounders, albeit dressed up differently:

> Cartwright, Papineau and Pearl are all in effect presenting...the argument that randomization controls for all possible confounders known and *unknown* [47].

In short, the link between randomization and "genuine" causes depends on the view that randomization rules out all confounders, whether they are known or unknown. Since randomization does not rule out all confounders, either probabilistic causality cannot require it, or we cannot establish probabilistic causes.

Perhaps more importantly, there is no reason for anyone involved in the EBM movement to take a stand on the rather obtuse philosophical debate on how probabilistic causes can be established.

CHAPTER 6

Questioning double blinding as a universal methodological virtue of clinical trials: resolving the Philip's paradox

. . . many investigators and readers delineate a randomized trial as high quality if it is "double-blind," as if double-blinding is the sine qua non of a randomized controlled trial. . . . A randomized trial, however, can be methodologically sound. . . and not be double-blind or, conversely, double-blind and not methodologically sound.

—K.F. Schulz & D.A. Grimes [222]

6.1 The problems with double masking as a requirement for clinical trial validity

Being "double blind" or "double masked," where neither the participants nor caregivers are aware of who gets the experimental treatment, is almost universally trumpeted as being a virtue of medical experiments. For example, the official EBM textbook states:

> Blinding is necessary to avoid patients' reporting of symptoms or their adherence to treatment being affected by hunches about whether

The Philosophy of Evidence-Based Medicine, First Edition. Jeremy Howick.
© 2011 Jeremy Howick. Published 2011 by Blackwell Publishing Ltd.

the treatment is effective. Similarly, blinding prevents the report or interpretation of symptoms from being affected by the clinician's or outcomes assessor's suspicions about the effectiveness of the study intervention [34].

Praise for double masking is not limited to EBM proponents. The US Food and Drug Administration (FDA) [254], systems for ranking the quality of evidence [19,21,255,256], prominent medical researchers [184,257), and medical statisticians [174,189] all explicitly claim that double blinding is a methodological virtue.

The view that double masking is useful has strong intuitive appeal: failure to maintain successful double masking leads to confounding. If an investigator is aware that particular participants are in the experimental arm of the trial, he or she may lavish more attention on them. The experimenter could also encourage them to remain in the trial, or adhere to the regimen. Indeed there is evidence that increased attention could have therapeutic benefits [258]. Similarly, if participants believe they are receiving the best treatment (as opposed to the placebo), then their knowledge that they are in the experimental arm could lead them not only to report better outcomes, but also to experience greater beneficial effects.

In spite of its appeal and widespread support, the view that double masking is valuable leads to the Philip's paradox [259] that our most dramatically effective treatments are not supportable by "best" (masked) evidence. Dramatically effective therapies, ranging from the Heimlich maneuver to unblock airways, external defibrillation to start a stopped heart, and epinephrine for anaphylactic shock, are so evidently effective that attempts to keep studies of such treatments "blind" or "masked" will inevitably fail. It seems strange, to say the very least, that an account of evidence should judge, *a priori*, that highly effective treatments can never be supported by "best evidence." Intuitively it would seem that they should receive much greater support from the evidence than do claims about treatments with only moderate effect sizes.

In this chapter I will argue that double masking does not always rule out confounding factors and hence that the Philip's paradox does not arise. To anticipate, I begin by clarifying what "double masking" means. Next, I explain why double masking is an instrumental good: it is valuable insofar as it rules out potential confounders arising from participant and caregiver knowledge of who receives the experimental intervention. The instrumental usefulness of double masking has two consequences. First, double masking must be successful in order to perform its intended function. Second, when the dramatic effects of the experimental intervention on the target disorder *cause* failure to successfully mask a study, subsequent participant and caregiver knowledge of who receives the experimental treatment does not give rise to confounding factors. The difference between what I call "benign" and "malicious" failure to maintain a successful double mask provides the basis for resolving the Philip's paradox.

6.2 The many faces of double masking: clarifying the terminology

Masking is the act of concealing the nature of the experimental intervention from one of the groups involved in the study. For example, in a single-masked randomized trial of vitamin C versus placebo as a cure for the common cold, the participants in the trial could be prevented from knowing whether they were taking the placebo or real vitamin C. This can be achieved by using a "vitamin C placebo" that is superficially indistinguishable from real vitamin C. Six groups involved in a trial are sometimes masked, namely participants, caregivers, data collectors, outcome evaluators, statisticians, and manuscript authors. The same person, or people, might, of course, be in more than one group. A caregiver might be in charge of allocation, dispensing the intervention, reporting outcomes, collecting data, evaluating outcomes, conducting the required statistical tests, and even authoring the manuscript. However, different groups *can* play these roles and even the same person could be masked at different stages of the study, and it is useful to distinguish them for purposes of analysis.

My use of the term "masked" instead of the more common "blind" requires some defence. The term "blind" is ambiguous in trials of blind people, and it is especially abhorred by researchers of eye disease [174]. Second, "masking" someone implies that the concealment procedure could be imperfect. As I will argue below, successful masking is inherently difficult to achieve. Third, the term "masking" is more in line with the historical meaning. Early trials that concealed the nature of the treatments from participants literally used masks [260].

A "double-masked" study is a study where at least two of the groups mentioned above are masked. Unfortunately, researchers rarely divulge *which* two, and this can be confusing. For example, Devereaux *et al.* found that a survey of 91 Canadian physicians interpreted "double masking" in 17 different ways, and a survey of 25 textbooks identified since 1990 provided nine definitions of "double masking." Just over one-third of the physician and textbook definitions characterized double masking as concealing knowledge from participants and caregivers. The remaining definitions included various combinations of two, three, and four masked groups. Because of this ambiguity, the CONSORT (Consolidated

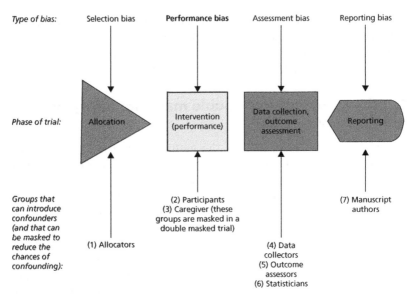

Figure 6.1 Various phases of a trial, types of bias introduced at each phase, and groups that can be masked at each phase to reduce the respective biases.

Standards of Reporting Trials) statement recommends identifying the particular groups that have been masked rather than using the terms "single masked," "double masked" or "triple masked" [255,261].

I will reserve the term "double masked" for trials that mask the participants and the caregivers. The rationale for my choice is twofold. First, "double masking" is most commonly used to describe trials where these two groups are masked. Second, the beliefs and expectations of only these two groups affects the *performance* phase of the trial after the intervention has been allocated and before the data have been gathered (Figure 6.1). My arguments about the qualified value of double masking (i.e. masking the participants and caregivers) do not bear on the importance of masking data collectors, outcome evaluators, statisticians, and manuscript authors (I will say more about masking these other groups in Chapter 12).

6.3 Confounders that arise from participant and caregiver knowledge

Recall from the introduction to Part II that a confounding factor is one that

1 potentially affects the outcome;

2 is unequally distributed between experimental and control groups; and

3 is unrelated to the experimental intervention.

Failure to mask participants and caregivers can lead to several confounders, including "belief" effects, "observer bias," concomitant medication, and drop-outs.

A participant's belief that she is being treated with an effective drug could, at least in theory, affect the outcome of interest. Innovative studies reveal how beliefs can have real effects. In one such study, Benedetti *et al.* [262] used four common painkillers – buprenorphine, tramadol, ketorolac, and metamizol – on a total of 278 patients who had undergone thoracic surgery for different pathological conditions. The postoperative patients were taken to have provided their informed consent when they were "told that they could receive either a painkiller or nothing depending on their postoperative state and that they will not necessarily be informed when any analgesic treatment will be started" [262]. The patients were then, of course unbeknownst to them, randomized into "overt" and "covert" groups with baseline factors such as sex, age, weight, and pain balanced. The "overt" group was treated by doctors who "gave the open drug at the bedside, telling them that the injection was a powerful analgesic and that the pain was going to subside in a few minutes" [262]. Then one dose of analgesic was administered every 15 minutes until a 50% reduction of pain (from baseline) was achieved for each patient. The "covert" group, on the other hand, had the analgesic delivered by a preprogrammed infusion machine (already attached to the patient for other reasons) without any doctor or nurse in the room. The pain reduction for both sets of patients was measured every 15 minutes on a 10-point subjective pain scale where 0 indicates no pain and 10 unbearable pain. Patients treated *covertly* required an average of 30% more analgesic than those treated overtly (*P*-values ranging from 0.02 to 0.007 depending on drug). This suggests that, at least for pain, patient beliefs that they are being treated by a "real" treatment can have relevant effects.

I will call the effects of knowledge that one is being treated with something one believes at least may be effective "belief effects" (sometimes called "expectation effects" or "conditioning effects" [262–264]. It is irrelevant for the purposes of my argument which term one prefers or how the effects are believed to arise.

Even in cases where beliefs might not have strong effects, participants' knowledge that they are receiving a "real" intervention may lead them to *report* that they feel better or recovered more quickly. Likewise, patients who believe they are receiving a mere placebo could drop out of the trial or seek outside treatments without informing the investigators. Differential drop-outs or rates of taking concomitant medication could confound the results of a study.

Caregiver knowledge can lead to a related set of confounding factors. A classic, though non-medical example of how caregiver knowledge may have effects is the Pygmalion experiment carried out by Robert Rosenthal and Lenore Jacobsen. (Pygmalion was the name of a Greek artist who sculpted a statue out of ivory and fell in love with it. Subsequently, because of the love lavished upon it, the statue allegedly came to life.)

In the spring of 1964, in a real public (state-funded) elementary school Rosenthal and Jacobsen call the Oak School (the real name is withheld), experimenters administered the "Harvard Test of Inflected Acquisition" to all (> 500) students in grades 1 to 5. Teachers were told that the test "predicts the likelihood that a child will show an inflection point or 'spurt' [point of rapid academic improvement] within the near future" [265]. Teachers administered the test, and two blind assessors scored them separately. The teachers were then given the names of the students who were most likely to "spurt." Teachers were told that the reason for divulging the names of the students was that it might interest them to know which students were likely to bloom, and were cautioned not to discuss the results with their pupils or the children's parents.

In fact the test was a standard IQ test, and the 20% of students who were predicted to "spurt" were chosen completely at random! After a year, the same IQ test was administered by the teachers and graded by independent, blind assessors. The top 20% of the students named by the test improved in all areas (including IQ) significantly more than the other students (Table 6.1).

The Oak School experiment suggests that teachers' expectations can have objective effects on student performance. More generally it suggests that *"one person's expectation for another person's behavior can quite unwittingly become a more accurate prediction simply for its having been made"* (italics original) [265].

Table 6.1 Mean gain in total IQ after One year by experimental- and control-group children in each of Six grades

Grade	Control		Experimental		Expectancy advantage	
	N	Gain	N	Gain	Iq Points	One-tailed *P* < 0.05
1	48	+12.0	7	+27.4	+15.4	0.002
2	47	+7.0	12	+16.5	+9.5	0.02
3	40	+5.0	14	+5.0	−0.0	
4	49	+2.2	12	+5.6	+3.4	
5	26	+17.5 (+)	9	+17.4 (−)	+0.0	
6	45	+10.7	11	+10.0	−0.7	
Total	255	+8.42	65	+12.22	+3.8	0.02

Recreated from table 7.1 in Rosenthal & Jacobson [265]. Note that the number of participants in the experimental group is not exactly 20% of the total. This is because "it was felt more plausible if each teacher did not have exactly the same number or percentage of her class listed" [265].

The mechanism of Pygmalion effects is not necessarily mysterious. A teacher, believing that a student was ready to "spurt," might pay special attention to that student which could easily translate into accelerated rates of improvement. At the same time, the scarce resources spent on the "spurters" are not "wasted" on those less likely to improve.

If there are Pygmalion effects in medicine, then if a caregiver believes that she is administering the best experimental treatment (as opposed to placebo) to a patient, she might treat that group differently, perhaps by providing a higher standard of care. Meanwhile, if the caregiver believed that a different patient was being given a placebo, she might not bother providing the highest quality of care – she might deem it not worthwhile, especially given that she has scarce resources to distribute amongst her many patients. Alternatively, a caregiver motivated by pity might bend over backwards and provide patients in the placebo arm with a higher quality of care. An obvious scenario where caregiver knowledge could have effects is if the caregiver has a personal or financial interest in showing that the experimental treatment works. The role of these personal or financial interests could be conscious or, more charitably, unconscious.

Moreover, if the caregiver is not successfully masked they could inform the participants (either directly or via "subtle cues") that they are taking the experimental therapy or placebo, which could cause the confounders introduced by participant knowledge to arise.

To sum up, failure to double mask a trial opens the door to several confounders that arise from participant and caregiver knowledge of who receives the experimental intervention. According to the methodological rule outlined in the introduction to Part II of this book, it would therefore appear that double masking increases the quality of a study. Importantly, however, double masking is an *instrumental* rather than *intrinsic* good: it is useful insofar as it rules out confounders. The instrumental value of double masking has two consequences: (i) in order to perform its intended function it must be successful; and (ii) it must actually rule out confounders to be useful.

6.4 The importance of *successful* double masking

Although current medical science often relies upon the double blind trial to determine the value of a medication, there is very little evidence that the double blind trial is blind for anybody, except those who read the report.

—P.G. Ney, C. Collins & C. Spensor [259]

One can attempt to keep a trial double masked by making the experimental and control therapy as outwardly indistinguishable as possible. For example, placebo pills should be the same color, weight, and taste as the real drug. If the control and experimental interventions are outwardly indistinguishable, participants and caregivers may not be able to detect whether they are taking the experimental therapy *at the start of the trial*. However, outwardly similar appearance is no guarantee that the trial will remain successfully double masked for the duration of the trial. For example, participants and caregivers are likely to identify experimental drugs that have a fishy taste, cause urine to turn blue, or produce recognizable side-effects. Clearly, if masking is unsuccessful, then confounders that arise from participant and caregiver knowledge are as worrisome as they would be if the trial was not double masked at all. If double masking is to be valuable it must perform its intended function: it must *successfully* keep participants and caregivers ignorant of whether they are taking the experimental intervention.

The success of masking at the end of the trial (or at some other suitable point) can be ascertained by asking participants whether or not they believe they received the experimental intervention. If the same proportion of participants in the control group believed they were taking the experimental intervention as those in the experimental group, we can safely assume that the trial was successfully double masked. Otherwise, there is (at least some degree of) evidence of "unmasking."

Unfortunately, the handful of empirical studies that have investigated the success of attempts to keep a trial double masked suggest that most fail. In 1986 Ney *et al.* [259] found that less than 5% of trials *described* as double masked actually performed tests to show the success of double masking. The authors provided some quantitative information about the reasons for the failure to keep trials successfully double masked:

> In assessing the effectiveness of penfluridal, the authors found sixteen of twenty five patients on active medication, had extrapyramidal side effects compared to three restless patients in the "placebo" group. In a study of amitriptyline, 45% of the patients dropped out of the active medication group because of side effects compared to 27% in the "placebo" group who dropped out because they were feeling no treatment effect. In this study the authors inferred the patients knew which group they were in although they did not check. In an investigation of the effects of intravenous cocaine the patients had an average increase of 48mmHg systolic blood pressure. There were many others of a similar nature where it was likely the patients were aware of the effect of the medication, and decided they were not on placebo [259].

The study by Ney *et al.* has been replicated more recently by research teams in Canada [266] and Scandinavia [267]. In the larger study,

Fergusson *et al.* [266] conducted a Medline search of randomized "pla-cebo"-controlled trials published from 1998 to 2001 in five top gen-eral medicine and four top psychiatry journals (*Journal of the American Medical Association, New England Journal of Medicine, The Lancet, British Medical Journal, Annals of Internal Medicine, Archives of General Psychiatry, Jour-nal of Clinical Psychiatry, British Journal of Psychiatry,* and *American Journal of Psychiatry*). Their search turned up a total of 473 medical and 192 psy-chiatry trials. From these they randomly selected 100 trials in each group. Nine of the randomly selected trials were excluded because they were not placebo-controlled despite being described as such; they ended up with 97 medical trials and 94 psychiatry trials. Of the 97 medical trials, only seven provided evidence of the success of double masking. Of these, only two reported that the masking was successful. Of the 94 psychiatry trials, eight reported evidence of testing for successful masking. Four of these reported that the masking was unsuccessful [266]. In short, there is evidence that masking is rarely tested for and, where tested for, rarely successful.

The problem with unsuccessful masking is well illustrated in a few studies that measured the difference in effects between trials employing "active" and those employing "normal" placebos. "Active"[4] placebos are not only sensibly indistinguishable from the test treatment, but also imitate some of the experimental treatment's side-effects [190–192]. Moncrieff and col-leagues found that active placebos reduce the apparent characteristic ben-efit of antidepressant drugs. In a related study, Kemp *et al.* [270] found a correlation between the apparent characteristic effects of schizophrenia drugs and the "strength" of the side-effects. The most plausible explana-tion for the increased effects of "active" placebos is that participants and caregivers correctly identify placebos that do not imitate any side-effects. This knowledge led to confounding beliefs and expectations regarding recovery.

Rather distressingly, there are good reasons to believe that successful double masking will remain elusive. To keep the trial successfully masked, the outward appearance, smell, taste, and side-effects of the experimental intervention must be mimicked by the control. Informed consent requires that participants are made aware of the nature of the experimental intervention, including its suspected benefits and side-effects. This means

---

[4]The choice of the term "active" [27,190,193,268,269] is rather unfortunate since all placebos are potentially active. However, I will not deviate from common usage and continue to use the term "active placebos" to denote placebos that have addi-tional ingredients that mimic some of the side-effects of the experimental therapy.

that a patient who experiences a particular side-effect might correctly deduce they are taking the experimental therapy rather than the placebo. To be sure, there is evidence that placebos can produce negative side-effects (*nocebo* effects) [271–274]. At the same time, nocebo effects seem to be less powerful than "non-placebo" effects [259].

One might be tempted to believe that the solution to unsuccessful masking is simply to increase the use of "active" placebos. While this will undoubtedly improve the success of masking, it is unlikely to solve the problem entirely because many side-effects are difficult to replicate without introducing further problems. For example, one side-effect of SSRIs is increased probability of sexual dysfunction. Even if a drug causing sexual dysfunction were added to the placebo, further complications would emerge. For one, it would have to be established that the ingredient added to the placebo in order to induce sexual dysfunction had no effects (either positive or negative) on depression, which would presumably require a separate study. These problems are compounded by the fact that most treatments have more than one side-effect. Moreover, it is unclear whether "active" placebos are ethical; participants in the control arm of a randomized trial receiving an "active" placebo would be experiencing some adverse effects and no potential benefit of the experimental treatment (see Chapter 8).

While worrisome even for drug trials, maintaining a successful double mask is amplified for non-drug treatments. For example, although "placebo"-controlled trials of surgical techniques have been performed [275–279], they are generally considered unethical, mostly because of the inherent risks involved even with placebo surgery [280]. More importantly, even if ethical, the surgeon performing the sham operation will (one hopes) be aware of whether he is performing real or sham surgery, which makes the attitudes of the surgeon a potential confounder. The only conceivable way to keep surgical trials double masked would be if the procedure were entirely mechanized. While robots sometimes assist physicians [281–284], they are not yet sophisticated enough to perform most operations on their own. Besides surgery, psychotherapy (or any form of "talking" therapy) and acupuncture cannot (at least not straightforwardly) be imitated by treatments that permit the trial to remain double masked.

To recap, unless successful, double masking does not rule out confounding factors that arise from participant and caregiver knowledge of who receives the experimental intervention.

Before examining the other consequence of the fact that double masking is an instrumental good, I will briefly discuss a practical problem with *testing* whether a trial has been successfully masked.

6.4.1 Problems, and a solution, to tests for successful masking

Sackett objects that the tests we use to measure successful masking can be confounded by "hunches about efficacy." The following anecdote illustrates just why.

> This dawned on our research group 30 years ago in a. . . trial of aspirin and sulfinpyrazone for preventing stroke in patients with transient ischaemic attacks (TIAs). At the end of the trial, but before we told them its results, study neurologists were asked to predict both the overall study results and the regimens for each of their patients. With four regimens, we would expect blind clinicians to guess the correct one for 25% of their patients. As it happened, they did statistically significantly worse than chance, correctly identifying regimens for only 18% of their patients! Our faulty reasoning was exposed when we examined their predictions of the overall study results: they had predicted that sulfinpyrazone was efficacious and aspirin was not, precisely the reverse of the trial's actual result. It then dawned on us that we were not testing our neurologists for blindness, but for their hunches about efficacy. When their patient had done well they tended to predict they were on (what they mistakenly thought was effective) sulfinpyrazone, and when they had done poorly, on "placebo" or (what they mistakenly thought was ineffective) aspirin [285].

In this example, the test for the success of masking indicated that masking was unsuccessful but in fact neurologists had *not* identified the experimental therapy (sulfinpyrazone) – they mistook it for aspirin. Had the test for successful masking been taken at face value, trialists might have mistakenly questioned the trial's result. In fact, the neurologists' hunches would have tended to make sulfinpyrazone appear even *less* effective than it actually was. Sackett concludes that

> [e]nd-of-trial tests for "blindness" can't be done with validity, because they can't distinguish blindness from hunches about efficacy. Moreover, although it often is appropriate to test regimens before a trial to be sure that they are indistinguishable, testing for blindness early in a trial, before any events and the consequent hunches have occurred, can't predict its status later in the trial [285].

As a result of Sackett's and others' [286] objections, the CONSORT group recently modified their guideline for the reporting of clinical trials by *omitting* the requirement to describe the method used for assessing the success of masking [261].

Rather than testing for the success of masking as a measure of whether confounding factors have been eliminated, Sackett suggests that we test directly for the presence of confounders that arise from unsuccessful masking. For example, whether patients have sought medication outside the trial can be measured by blood or urine tests (Sackett did this in his TIA trial), and biased reporting can be ruled out by employing masked outcome evaluators. We might also measure the prevalence of various side-effects in different arms of a trial (Ney *et al.* did this in their review described above). If certain recognizable side-effects are far more prevalent in the experimental arm of a trial, then we might suspect that the masking was unsuccessful and worry that the study had come unmasked and worry about potential confounding. (It is worth mentioning that the authors of the latest CONSORT statement do not replace the suggestion to report the success of masking with Sackett's suggestions to directly measure the presence of confounders that arise due to lack of masking.)

Sackett is correct that tests for the success of masking can be confounded by hunches about efficacy, and that the *purpose* of testing for the success of masking – to verify whether certain confounding factors have been ruled out – can be (at least partly) achieved by other means. Perhaps most importantly, Sackett's objection highlights the problem of accepting the results of *any* test without pausing to think.

At the same time, Sackett is too quick to dismiss tests for successful masking. It is possible to discover whether a test for the success of blinding has been confounded by hunches about efficacy. We might simply ask physicians (and patients) why they believed they were (or were not) in the experimental arm of the study. Even in the TIA study, Sackett and his team were able to find out (presumably by asking) why physicians believed that certain patients were taking sulfinpyrazone. Tests for successful masking could be expanded to include questions about why the participants or caregivers believed they were (or were not) in the experimental group. While in theory caregivers or participants could answer these questions inaccurately [286], empirical evidence suggests that in practice accurate answers are possible [266,267].

The second problem is that the alternative strategies Sackett proposes have problems of their own. For example, while trialists can measure whether participants "cheated" by taking *some* other medications, other factors are far more difficult to measure. At least for certain outcomes (such as depression and pain), whether participants feel better, take more exercise, or sleep better can affect outcomes but are far more difficult to measure objectively.

Finally, tests for successful masking and measuring for the presence of confounders directly can mutually reinforce one another to verify whether confounding has been eliminated. Tests for successful masking, even in their modified form, do not involve much more work and, provided they are interpreted sensibly, can provide useful information. More generally, as Shapiro notes "[i]t seems contrary to an evidence based approach to avoid obtaining data because we have to struggle with its interpretation" [287].

Indeed, tests for successful masking are useful even when they have been confounded by hunches about efficacy. In the TIA study Sackett cites, neurologists tended to believe that patients who recovered successfully had been prescribed sulfinpyrazone. These differential beliefs could have confounded the study in any of the various ways mentioned earlier in this chapter. For example, the neurologists could have reported the outcomes differently, subtly encouraged patients taking what they believed to be aspirin or placebo to seek outside help, or compound the problem by conveying their beliefs to the patients. These confounders would have tended to detract from any effects of sulfinpyrazone and provide an inaccurate estimate of its effects.

Meanwhile, tests for successful masking could be buttressed by testing for confounders that arise from unsuccessful double masking that Sackett recommends.

Perhaps most importantly for the purposes of this chapter, practical problems with current tests for the success of masking do not affect my argument that in order to perform its function, double-masking must be *successful*. Even Sackett would presumably agree: his objection is to practical problems with current tests for the success of masking. Indeed the goal of measuring whether a trial has been confounded is perhaps best achieved with a combination of testing for the success of masking *and* measuring for the presence of other confounders.

6.5 One (and a half) solutions to the Philip's paradox

The Philip's paradox arises from the view that double masking increases the quality of the trial (by reducing confounding). I will argue that double masking does not increase the quality of the study where effects are dramatically apparent and hence that the Philip's paradox does not arise. There is also a sense in which the Philip's paradox can be resolved by appeal to the rule of evidence outlined in the previous chapter that the essential feature of good evidence is that the effect size outweighs the combined effects of plausible confounders.

6.5.1 (Half) of a resolution to the Philip's paradox: sometimes effect size swamps the potentially confounding results of failure to mask

Sometimes participant and caregiver beliefs may not have important effects [168,169]. More importantly, potential confounders ruled out by successful double masking would be unlikely to account for dramatic effects. Acute appendicitis or meningitis might well be influenced by the potential confounders ruled out by successful masking, but not enough to account for the dramatic effect of appendectomies and antibiotics for meningitis. In these cases, the effect size swamps the potentially confounding influence of the factors that arise from participant or caregiver knowledge of who receives the experimental intervention. Hence, according to the rule of evidence suggested last chapter, we could argue that the quality of the study is not reduced by (relatively unimportant) confounding factors when the effect size is sufficiently dramatic. In practice, of course, this is what happens. When appraising the quality of evidence for therapy, the EBM movement allows for non-randomized studies to count as high quality when "the treatment effect described in the non-randomized trial is so huge that you can't imagine it could be a false-positive study" [32]. However, there is a more fundamental resolution to the Philip's paradox.

6.6 The full solution to the Philip's paradox: challenging the view that double masking rules out confounding factors when treatments are evidently dramatic

In some cases participants taking the experimental treatment *know* they are taking the experimental treatment but such knowledge does not introduce confounders. Imagine we conducted a double-masked trial of epinephrine versus placebo (this would *not* be ethical – I use the hypothetical example for explanatory purposes only) for anaphylactic shock. The effects of the treatment, often making an unconscious person conscious, would be so apparent that attempts to maintain double masking would fail. Patients and caregivers would realize which injection was real epinephrine and which was the placebo, and the potential confounders that arise from such knowledge could well occur. For example, patients and caregivers would recognize the experimental treatment and believe in its effectiveness, while those assigned to the placebo group would undoubtedly drop out immediately to seek concomitant medication. However, these *potential* confounders do not satisfy the third condition for being a confounder: they are related to the experimental intervention (Figure 6.2). When failure to

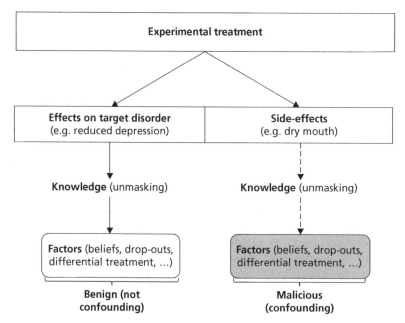

Figure 6.2 The difference between confounding and non-confounding factors arising from failure to maintain successful double masking.

successfully double mask a trial results from the dramatic effects of a treatment, the resulting factors arising from participant and caregiver knowledge are not confounding.

But we must be more precise: beliefs that arise due to the side-effects of the treatment (as opposed to the effects on the target disorder) are also related to the intervention yet they *are* confounding. This was apparent in the trials contrasting active with standard placebos used in depression trials cited earlier [29,190–192]. Here failure to successfully mask a trial was caused by the (side-effects of the) experimental treatment and we would like to call the factors that arose due to participant and caregiver knowledge confounding.

The difference, of course, is that in one case the knowledge arose from the treatment's effects on the target disorder, while in the other they arose from the side-effects. With that in mind, the third condition for being considered a confounding factor must be modified. In order to be considered confounding, a factor must:

3' be unrelated to the positive characteristic effects of the experimental treatment on the target disorder (as opposed to side-effects).

In short, unmasking caused by side-effects, ineffective attempts to make the experimental and control treatments appear similar, or outright cheating, introduces confounding and is what I shall refer to as *malicious* unmasking (see Figure 6.2). On the other hand, unmasking caused by the dramatic characteristic effects of the treatment on the target disorder will not cause confounders and is what I shall call *benign* unmasking (see Figure 6.2). Considering the causes of unmasking (benign or malicious) provides us with a way to distinguish between trials where successful double masking is a methodological virtue and those where it adds no value (or even detracts from a trial's value). The Philip's paradox is resolved by noting that in cases where the dramatic positive characteristic effects of a treatment on the target disorder prevent the trial from being double masked, the failure to successfully mask does not detract from the quality of the trial. This is because no confounders have been introduced as a result of subsequent participant and caregiver knowledge. In fact, we might reward a trial where failure to maintain a successful double mask has been caused by the dramatic effects of a treatment.

I have, of course, been discussing the simple case where unmasking arises due to either the characteristic effects on the target disorder or some less benign reason. In practice the reasons for failure to successfully mask could be mixed or even difficult to ascertain. More theoretical and empirical work is required to adjudicate in these more complex cases.

6.7 Double masking is valuable unless the treatment effects are evidently dramatic, hence the Philip's paradox does not arise

Double masking is instrumentally valuable because it can reduce confounding during the performance phase of the trial including belief effects, drop-outs, and concomitant medication. Hence double masking is widely regarded as a methodological virtue of clinical trials. Given that randomized trials but not observational studies can employ double masking, this provides a further potential benefit of randomized trials over observational studies. However, the view that double masking adds methodological value leads to the Philip's paradox that dramatically effective treatments cannot be supported by double masked, and hence "best" evidence. The paradox arises from a false premise that double masking always increases the quality of a trial (by reducing confounding). The paradox can also be resolved by noting that where treatment effects are dramatic, the effects of confounders arising from participant and caregiver knowledge are relatively unimportant.

The results of this chapter have implications for the debate surrounding the superiority of randomized trials over observational studies. Recall that randomized trials (especially those that employ concealed allocation) are less likely to suffer from allocation bias and patient preference bias than observational studies. However, randomized trials can be (but are not necessarily) conducted in double-masked conditions while observational studies cannot. If double masking were a universal virtue of studies, then double-masked randomized trials would have a further benefit over observational studies. In this chapter I found that double masking usually adds methodological value and will therefore usually provide double-masked randomized trials with a methodological advantage over observational studies. However in some exceptional cases, namely when effect sizes are dramatic and apparent, double masking does not add methodological value and will therefore not increase the relative advantage of randomized trials over observational studies.

In the next chapter I will consider the next potential benefit of randomized trials over observational studies, namely their practically unique ability to employ "placebo" controls.

CHAPTER 7

Placebo controls: problematic and misleading baseline measures of effectiveness

Is there a need to control the "placebo" in "placebo" controlled trials?

—A.J. DE CRAEN ET AL. [288]

The perfect placebo, therefore, would be one which would mimic exactly all qualities and effects of the drug under study except for the effect in question. Obviously, in many cases the achievement of the perfect "placebo" is an actual impossibility.

—L. LASAGNA [249]

7.1 The need to control the placebo

To evaluate whether "placebo" or "active" controlled randomized trials provide better evidence, we need to understand what placebo controls *are*. As we shall see, the label *placebo control* is used to describe a plethora of different treatments, ranging from longer consultations and sugar pills to acupuncture using needles that do not penetrate the skin and supervised flexibility. Moreover, some control therapies labeled "placebos" have ingredients that are not, on close scrutiny, placebic. In one example, olive oil was used in placebo capsules for trials of cholesterol-lowering agents before there was evidence that olive oil reduced cholesterol:

> several early papers exploring the use of cholesterol-lowering agents
> to curb heart disease did in fact name the placebos used: olive oil in

The Philosophy of Evidence-Based Medicine, First Edition. Jeremy Howick.
© 2011 Jeremy Howick. Published 2011 by Blackwell Publishing Ltd.

one case, and corn oil in another. Mono- and poly-unsaturates such as olive oil and corn oil are now widely known to decrease low-density lipoproteins, so that with hindsight these agents may not have been inert with respect to the outcome studied. Indeed, it was noted in one such study that the rate of cardiac mortality was lower in the "placebo" group than expected [289].

This suggests that use of the ambiguous term "placebo control" can have serious consequences for the appraisal and interpretation of randomized trials: we need standards for placebo controls. Many will dismiss my concerns here as pedantic and assert that placebo controls are simply "inactive" or "non-specific" [290] substances that are capable of making participants believe that they might be taking the "real" treatment. But these characterizations are grossly misleading [264,291]. There are currently no known substances that are completely physiologically inert although they could be inactive in a particular regard; in at least some cases placebos *are* active and moreover their effects can be quite specific [291,292]. Indeed recent studies using functional magnetic resonance imaging and positron emission tomography have revealed (specific!) mechanisms of action for both placebo and nocebo (negative placebo side-effects) analgesia [274,293–298].

Others associate placebo effects with beliefs and expectations. While beliefs and expectations are some of the factors placebo controls should control for, it is a mistake to assume that controlling for beliefs and expectations is a sufficient condition for legitimacy of placebo controls. Someone might believe that a pill containing olive oil was the real cholesterol-lowering drug but this would not mean that such a pill was a legitimate placebo control.

One plausible reason for the failure to set standards for placebo controls is that the placebo itself has resisted adequate conceptualization. None of the many attempts to define the placebo [290,291,299,300] has won widespread acceptance. The failure to adequately define "placebo," and the subsequent lack of standards for placebo controls, has led researchers to adopt questionable strategies when estimating the placebo effect. For instance, Hrobjartsson and Gøtzsche [168] characterize placebos "practically as an intervention labeled as such in the report of a clinical trial." However, as the example of olive oil placebos illustrates, allowing any treatment labeled as a placebo control in a clinical trial to count as a placebo invites inaccurate conclusions about a treatment's effects.

My main thesis here is that in spite of any difficulties in defining the placebo *per se* it is both possible and desirable to set standards for what I will call *legitimate placebo controls*. A legitimate placebo control is one that contains all and only the *characteristic* features of the experimental therapy. With the standards for legitimacy at hand, there are good reasons to believe legitimate placebo controls are far rarer than is commonly believed. However, the precise extent of the problem with illegitimate placebo controls is currently impossible to gauge because placebo controls are almost never described in sufficient detail to judge their legitimacy. I conclude with a suggestion that the label "placebo" be replaced, or at least accompanied by a detailed description of the treatment employed. Placebo controls are best conceptualized as treatments in their own right [301–303].

7.2 Legitimate placebo controls

Let us examine the "placebo" somewhat more critically, however, since it and "double blind" have reached the status of fetishes in our thinking and literature. The automatic aura of Respectability, Infallibility, and Scientific Savoir-faire which they possess for many can be easily shown to be undeserved in certain circumstances.

—L. LASAGNA [249]

Legitimate 'placebo' controls are the same as the experimental treatment but are missing only the characteristic features. More specifically, a treatment is a legitimate placebo control if, and only if, it satisfies the following conditions:

1 The placebo control contains all the relevant non-characteristic features of the test treatment *t*, to the same degree that they are present in the experimental treatment process.
2 The placebo control has no additional relevant features over and above the non-characteristic features of the experimental treatment.

Even treatments not thought of as complex have several components. For instance, treatment of depression with Prozac therapy involves ingestion of fluoxetine hydrochloride (in certain doses at certain times), ingestion of the other ingredients contained in the pill and the pill casing, the liquid with which the pill is swallowed, as well as the beliefs and expectations that are aroused by a prescription for Prozac, and perhaps many other features. Hence, patients never receive Prozac in isolation, but rather they receive a "treatment process involving Prozac," or "Prozac therapy" for short. The "characteristic" feature of treatment for depression involving Prozac is the fluoxetine hydrochloride – everything else is "non-characteristic."

A placebo-controlled trial estimates the effects of the characteristic features by subtracting the average effect in the placebo group (which should involve the effects of all and only the non-characteristic features) from the average effect of the experimental treatment (the effects of the characteristic plus non-characteristic features) (Figure 7.1).

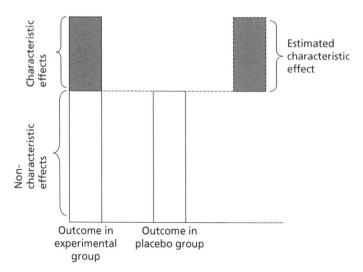

Figure 7.1 How placebo-controlled trials are supposed to provide a measure of the "characteristic" effects of a medical intervention.

If the placebo control is missing some relevant non-characteristic features of the experimental treatment (if the first condition for legitimacy is violated), then any observed difference will be augmented by an amount equivalent to the effects (if any) of the missing non-characteristic features (Figure 7.2). On the other hand, if the placebo control treatment process contains more than the non-characteristic features of the experimental treatment process, the apparent benefit of the characteristic features will be diminished by an amount equivalent to the effects (if any) of the additional features (Figure 7.3).

7.3 How placebo controls often violate the first condition for legitimacy

At first glance it might appear as though drug placebo controls easily satisfy the first condition for legitimacy. After all participants are simply treated with pills (or liquids) that look like the real drug but do not contain the characteristic chemical. The chemical is usually replaced with a supposedly innocent substance such as lactose. (Sometimes the characteristic chemical does not account for a substantial amount of the real pill's mass, in which case the real pill will contain a bulking agent already and nothing needs to be added to the placebo.) Such a placebo control treatment process might have an additional feature (lactose), but it does not appear to be missing

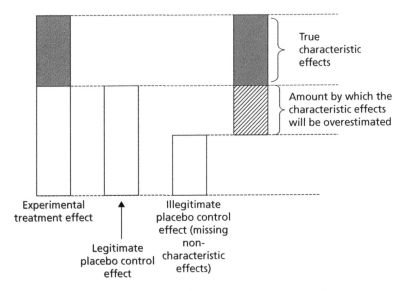

Figure 7.2 An illegitimate placebo control that leads to an overestimation of the apparent characteristic benefit of the experimental intervention.

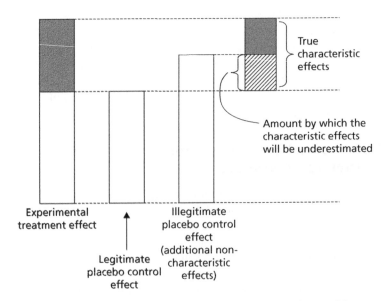

Figure 7.3 An illegitimate placebo control that leads to an underestimate of the apparent characteristic benefit of the experimental intervention.

anything. (I shall address the potential problems that arise with the introduction of replacement substances below.)

But if the control therapy does not induce the same degrees of belief or expectation as the experimental therapy, then the apparent characteristic benefit of the experimental treatment will be exaggerated by an amount equivalent to the effects (if any) of the reduction (or, in some cases, increase [285]) in expectation or belief (see Figure 7.2). For example, imagine a placebo-controlled trial of Prozac therapy for depression where the experimental group received real Prozac pills with "PROZAC" written on them, while the control group received lactose pills with the word "PLACEBO" written on them. Participants who believed they were being treated with a mere placebo would be likely to have lower expectations about their chances of recovery compared with the participants receiving real Prozac.[5]

Here the placebo control therapy would be missing some degree of expectation that was induced by the experimental therapy, and therefore might be illegitimate. The different levels of expectation rather than any potential effects of fluoxetine hydrochloride might explain any observed difference between treatment with real and placebo Prozac therapy.

The easy way to make sure that expectations are the same in experimental and control groups is to blind (or mask) the participants for the duration of the trial. We saw in Chapter 6, however, that successful double masking is far more difficult to achieve than many suppose. The placebo control treatment process for an intervention whose side-effects are not easily imitated or whose characteristic features have distinctive smells or tastes will often be identifiable as placebos and therefore fail to induce the same participant or dispensing physician expectations.

If successful masking is a condition for placebo control legitimacy – and trials are rarely successfully masked – then the placebo group will not be legitimate since it will be lacking the same expectations regarding recovery as the experimental group.

Skeptics about placebo effects would no doubt object that expectations rarely have effects [168,169]. For instance, a patient's expectation of

---

[5]This may not always be the case. In an interesting study of neurotic patients [304], researchers examined the effect of placebos delivered in open (unblinded) conditions, i.e. they told the patients that they were delivering a placebo. They found that these patients were responsive to placebo even though they were informed that they were being given a placebo. However, the study was quite small and, perhaps more relevantly, the patients (because they were neurotic) did not believe that they had been given placebos!.

receiving an appendectomy for acute appendicitis could have greater effects than her expectation of receiving "placebo" surgery, but the effects are likely to be unimportant relative to the characteristic effectiveness of appendectomies. If the lower degree of expectations introduced by unsuccessful masking are ineffective, then failure to successfully implement masking will not threaten the legitimacy of the placebo control. However, we also saw from Chapter 6 that different expectations and beliefs, even if not directly effective, can introduce other differences between the placebo and experimental groups. A participant who is aware that he is in the control group (and hence that he is being withheld the experimental treatment) might drop out of the trial, or (which is worse for the study although possibly better for the patient) covertly seek "real" treatment outside the trial. If the participants taking the placebo control receive outside treatment, then there will be a further difference between their therapy and the treatment process administered to the experimental group, rendering the average placebo control treatment process illegitimate. In sum, failure to successfully mask participants and dispensers can violate the first condition for legitimacy of the placebo control even if beliefs and expectations have not significant effects.

7.4 How placebo controls often violate the second condition for legitimacy

A treatment could be delivered in successfully double-masked conditions but contain more than the non-characteristic features of the experimental treatment. The characteristic chemical of the experimental treatment will usually have to be replaced with some other substance. For instance, a Prozac placebo pill might replace fluoxetine hydrochloride with lactose. Because the replacement substance is not supposed to have effects on the target disorder, it will not render the placebo control treatment process illegitimate. Yet, as the earlier example of olive oil used in placebo controls for cholesterol-lowering drugs suggests, apparently innocent replacement substances sometimes have effects on the target disorder being studied. In another example the sweetness of the liquids in which antitussive drugs were administered was found to account for a significant portion of the observed effect of the experimental treatment [305,306]. If the placebo control treatment involved more sweet liquid (to replace the missing characteristic antitussive compound) than the experimental treatment process, then the placebo control will be more effective than the non-characteristic features of experimental treatment.

The extent of the problem with placebo controls which have additional substances that threaten legitimacy is currently unknown because placebo ingredients are rarely divulged. In a recent study, Golomb *et al.* [301] found that randomized trials involving placebo tablets divulged the placebo ingredients, while less than 10% of trials involving non-tablet placebos did so. Even if the additional feature does not have *direct* effects on the target disorder, it could, in some cases, lead to the unmasking of the participants, in which case they might render the placebo control treatment process illegitimate.

The problems for constructing legitimate placebo controls are more pronounced for complex treatments. For example, although placebo-controlled trials of surgical techniques have been performed [275–279], they are generally considered unethical, mostly because of the inherent risks involved with any surgery [280]. Even if they were ethical, the surgeon performing the sham operation will (one hopes) be aware of whether he is performing real or sham surgery and therefore impossible to successfully double mask. This undermines the legitimacy of most placebo controls used in surgical trials. The only way to keep surgical trials double masked would be if the procedure were entirely mechanized. Although robots sometimes assist physicians [281–284], they are not yet sophisticated enough to perform operations on their own. I will now illustrate the special difficulty with constructing legitimate placebo controls for these more complex treatments with case studies of exercise and acupuncture trials.

7.5 Special problem for constructing placebos for complex treatments: case studies of exercise and acupuncture

7.5.1 Illegitimate exercise placebos

Assume that the features (both non-characteristic and characteristic) of an extended program of exercise include at least the following:
1 belief that one is being treated with exercise;
2 participant/investigator (fitness trainer or advisor) interaction;
3 other "psychological" benefits of exercise (distraction from daily routine and worry, the sense of achievement and social interactions);
4 increased metabolic rate;
5 increased body temperature;
6 increased heart rate for some prolonged period of time;
7 increased endorphin and epinephrine levels caused by exercise.
One might take increased endorphin and epinephrine levels (factor 7) as characteristic of exercise therapy for depression [307,308]. Although this feature is conceptually distinguishable, it would be difficult, if not

impossible, to design a control treatment that contained all the other features of exercise less the increased endorphin and epinephrine levels.

Recognizing that identifying and isolating all but the non-characteristic
features of exercise is difficult or impossible, researchers have used control
therapies that are quite different from exercise therapy, including supervised relaxation [309] and supervised flexibility [310] and called them
placebo controls for exercise. I will contend that these control therapies are
not legitimate placebo controls for exercise therapy.

In the more recent study, low and high "doses" of exercise (each spread
out over three or five sessions per week) were compared with exercise placebo (supervised flexibility) for the treatment of major depressive disorder
[311]. The investigators randomized 80 participants to receive one of five
treatments for 12 weeks. The primary outcome measure was a change in
the 17-point Hamilton Rating Scale for Depression (HRSD17)[6] score from
baseline to 12 weeks. Blind assessors measured the HRSD17 scores each
week.

The main finding of the study was that a treatment process involving the
higher dose of exercise reduced the scores on the HRSD by an average of
47%. The treatment process involving a low dose of exercise reduced the
scores by an average of 30%, which was similar to the "placebo" treatment
process, which reduced the scores by an average of 29%.

However, there are several reasons to doubt whether supervised flexibility
is a legitimate exercise placebo for the treatment of depression. Firstly, the
placebo control treatments did not permit the trial to remain double masked
and therefore did not include any potential effects of expectation of taking
real exercise. Obviously, participants in the placebo group deduced that they
were in the placebo group. Both participants and investigators supervising
the intervention could have had different beliefs about the potency of each
intervention. Most likely, the belief that more intense exercise might be
more effective was disproportionately present in the treatment groups, while
the belief that flexibility was ineffective was disproportionately present in
the placebo control group. This means that the expectation effect could have
been stronger in the experimental groups and lowest in the placebo group.

---

[6]The HRSD17 [312] measures severity of depressive symptoms. It is a question-
naire with 17 questions that ask patients to rate themselves on a 3- or 5-point scale
(depending on the question) for symptoms such as insomnia, anxiety, depression,
and guilt. A score of 10–13 points (out of a possible 69) is taken as evidence that
the patient is considered mildly depressed; a score of 14–17 points, the patient is
considered mild to moderately depressed; a score above 17 points, the patient is
considered to be severely depressed. The HRSD17 has been widely used to measure
depressive symptoms since the 1960s.

If participant expectations have effects, and in the treatment of depression it is likely that they do [168,169], then the placebo treatment was missing a non-characteristic feature of treatment with the experimental intervention. This is sufficient to question the legitimacy of the placebo control. The placebo control treatment processes also omitted several other features of exercise therapy, including sustained increased heart rate.

Supervised flexibility also might have had *additional* features that could be characteristic for depression and hence violated the second condition for placebo control legitimacy. Yoga, for example, which may be little more than flexibility exercises used in trials of exercise, has been shown in at least one trial to reduce the symptoms of depression on the HRSD [313]. Likewise, relaxation (used in other "placebo"-controlled trials of exercise) might also have characteristic effects for depression. Exercise has been linked to the relaxation response in laboratory animals [314]. Benson's bestseller, *The Relaxation Response*, first published in 1975 and reissued in 2000, claims that relaxing for as little as 10 minutes per day can have a positive impact on depression. If it is true that flexibility or relaxation has effects over and above the non-characteristic effects of exercise, then they are illegitimate placebo controls. I am not of course making any claims about the potency of supervised flexibility for depression, only pointing to the possibility that flexibility and relaxation may have effects on depression that are greater than the non-characteristic effects of exercise *per se*.

It could be that the potential effects of the missing features (beliefs and expectations) and the potential effects of the additional features cancel out. But this would be highly unlikely, and moreover until this has been established we must refrain from deeming these exercise placebo controls as legitimate.

7.5.2 Illegitimate acupuncture placebos

Derived from traditional Chinese medicine, acupuncture is a form of treatment for various disorders that involves insertion of fine needles into particular points in the body known as *Qi* (pronounced "chee") or "acupuncture points." The needles are very thin and usually penetrate to a depth of 5–40 mm (¼ to ¾ of an inch) depending on the location of the point. The penetration of the needles into the skin is often barely perceptible. The FDA in the USA has removed its "experimental" label from acupuncture needles, and the National Institute for Health and Clinical Excellence (NICE) in the UK recommends acupuncture as an established treatment for some disorders, especially those involving pain. Yet it has proven difficult to design a placebo control treatment to be used in acupuncture trials until very recently.

One device touted as a placebo or "sham" acupuncture procedure involves the Streitberger needle [315]. This is a blunt needle embedded in a moveable shaft. When the blunt needle is pressed on the skin, the shaft moves and makes it appear as though the needle penetrates the skin. In order to hold the Streitberger needle in place, plastic rings are taped to the patient's skin at the acupuncture points. (To maintain the deception, the rings are also used for the real acupuncture in trials.) Some researchers claim that the sham needle is "validated," by which they mean a trial involving treatment with the sham device is capable of remaining successfully masked.

Yet it is unclear whether the sham device is a legitimate placebo control for acupuncture for several reasons. First, it is unclear whether the sham needle is, as some of its proponents claim, capable of being delivered in successfully double-masked conditions. The studies Kaptchuk *et al.* cite as evidence for validation provide only conditional support for the view that the Streitberger needle is indistinguishable from real acupuncture. The first study [315] asked patients to guess whether they felt any painful penetration of the needles, and they found no statistically significant difference in the subjective measures of pain between groups. However, more of those in the "real" acupuncture group felt a dull pain (54 of 60) than those in the placebo group (47 of 60). In the conclusion the authors claimed "acupuncture seems to be a little more painful than [and hence perhaps distinguishable from] 'placebo' needling" [315]. The second study [316] merely refers to the previous study and does not contain any new data. The third study [317] found evidence that participants could not distinguish the amount of penetration achieved by the placebo and real acupuncture, but they found that 40% of participants thought that the placebo acupuncture was different (in some unspecified way) from the real acupuncture. White *et al.* [317] conclude that the sham device does not permit the trial to remain successfully masked:

> If a prerequisite [for validation] of a "placebo" is that it is indistinguishable from the real treatment, then the fact that nearly 40% of subjects did not find that the two interventions were similar, however, raises some concerns. . .if this were a drug trial, would we be happy if 40% did not find the intervention to be similar. . .? [317].

Moreover, acupuncture *practitioners* are aware of whether they are using the Streitberger needle or real acupuncture, and could reveal, either directly or inadvertently, knowledge of who is taking the experimental treatment to the participants in a trial.

In short, it is questionable whether treatment with the sham device is truly "validated" (capable of being delivered in successfully masked conditions).

More importantly, validation is an insufficient condition for legitimacy. Besides being able to induce the same level of beliefs and expectations, a legitimate placebo control must *not* contain any of the characteristic features of the experimental treatment.

Indeed, there is considerable controversy surrounding the claim that the Streitberger needle is devoid of all characteristic features of real acupuncture [318–323]. To evaluate the controversy it is useful to note the features of acupuncture therapy which *might* play a role in outcome.

1 Patients' and practitioners' beliefs about, attitude towards, and expectations of needling and acupuncture.
2 The acupuncture consultation.
3 General physiological effects of needle insertion (anywhere in the body, not at the "acupuncture" points indicated by the relevant theory of acupuncture).
4 The (putative) effects of appropriate needle stimulation at the correct location.
5 The physiological effects of (acu)pressure.
6 The (putative) effects of (acu)pressure *at the correct location*.

If we bracket the problem that treatment with the Streitberger needle is distinguishable (at least to the practitioners) from real acupuncture, then Streitberger needle therapy controls for the fourth feature listed above (appropriate needle stimulation at the correct location). Yet there is a difference between a control treatment that controls for all but *one* feature and a control treatment that controls for *all* the non-characteristic features. To illustrate just why, consider co-amilofruse, the generic name for a drug that contains two agents known to have positive (non-placebo) effects on hypertension and edema, namely amiloride and frusemide. If our control treatment were identical to real co-amilofruse, apart from the fact that it was missing amiloride (but contained frusemide), then it would accurately measure the effects of amiloride. However, to say that such a control treatment was a legitimate placebo would be mistaken since the 'placebo' contained frusemide. To test whether co-amilofruse was more effective than a placebo, our control treatment should of course contain *neither* amiloride nor frusemide.

One might wish, of course, to measure the effects of each potential characteristic feature. In our example amiloride and frusemide would be separately evaluated and the component effects could then be added together to determine the overall effect. However, there are at least two problems with this approach. First, the characteristic features could interact making it difficult to predict their combined effect by adding their individual effects (see next chapter). Second, it is often impossible in practice to separate the various characteristic features.

The first reason to *suspect* that sham acupuncture might not be a legitimate placebo control is that the sham needles appear to be more effective than placebo pills and even conventional therapy. In a different study employing treatment with the sham needle, Kaptchuk *et al.* [324] found that treatment with the Streitberger needle was more effective than placebo pills for treatment of persistent upper extremity pain due to repetitive use. In the study of 270 participants, they compared one trial of real acupuncture therapy versus sham acupuncture (involving the Streitberger needle), and another of amitriptyline therapy versus placebo pill therapy. The authors conclude: "A validated sham acupuncture device has a greater '*placebo*' effect on subjective outcomes than oral 'placebo' pills" (my emphasis) [324].

Another study suggested that sham acupuncture is more effective even than other non-placebo drug therapies. In the German Acupuncture Trials (GERAC), acupuncture placebo[7] outperformed conventional therapy (biweekly consultations with physicians or physiotherapists who administered exercise, physiotherapy, and non-steroidal anti-inflammatory drugs or NSAIDs) for persistent lower back pain [325]. The primary outcomes were subjective measures of pain, i.e. rankings on scales where 10 indicated excruciating pain and 0 no pain. Successful treatment response after 6 months was defined as 33% improvement or better on the pain scales [325]. The response rate after 6 months, which was assessed by masked investigators, showed that 47.6% of the participants in the real acupuncture group, 44.2% in the sham acupuncture group, and 27.4% in the conventional therapy group recovered.

The difference between real and sham acupuncture in the GERAC trial was not statistically significant, but both real and sham acupuncture therapy were significantly more effective than conventional therapy. It is also relevant, although Haake *et al.* do not mention it, that there is considerable evidence that conventional therapy is better than a placebo pill. NSAIDs, which formed part of the conventional therapy, are more effective than treatment with NSAID placebos for lower back pain [326–328]. The results are best understood with the aid of a diagram (Figure 7.4).

---

[7]GERAC used a sham procedure that was different from the Streitberger needle. In the GERAC trial, the "placebo" needle penetrated the skin but avoided all known Qi points. What is relevant for present purposes is not an evaluation of whether the GERAC placebo was legitimate, but rather the fact that it was more effective than conventional therapy.

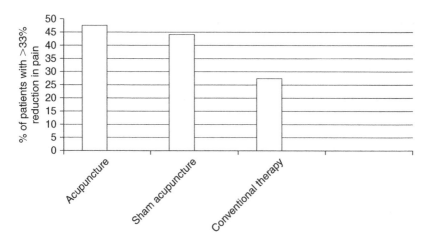

Figure 7.4 The different effects of different placebo treatments.

The trials indicating that acupuncture placebos are more effective than pill placebos reveal how confusing placebo-controlled trials can be. Besides being vague and imprecise, using the same label ("placebo control") to describe these diverse treatments with very different effects can be misleading. One treatment, say acupuncture, might fail to demonstrate superiority to a placebo in one trial, while another treatment, say ibuprofen, might demonstrate statistically significant and clinically relevant superiority to a (different) placebo in a different trial, and patients, clinicians, and policy-makers alike could easily fall into the trap of concluding that ibuprofen is more effective than acupuncture. Yet such a conclusion could be false and misleading because the non-characteristic effects of the various placebos might be different.

This brings us to the question of whether the Streitberger needle is in fact an illegitimate placebo control for acupuncture therapy, or simply an especially effective placebo. Although Kaptchuk prefers the latter interpretation, I will argue that the former interpretation is more plausible. To begin, there is independent evidence that acupressure is effective for pain relief [329–331]. I will not discuss this literature here, but only note that it is not *prima facie* obvious that acupressure is non-characteristic for treatment of pain. If it should be classified as characteristic, the Streitberger needle violates the second condition for legitimacy.

To make matters more complex, it is often argued that the acupuncture consultation (which is often much longer than a conventional consultation) should be classified as characteristic [332]. It is certainly true that longer consultations can have relevant positive effects. In yet another interest-ing study that we will examine in more detail in Chapter 11, Kaptchuk compared placebo acupuncture (involving the Streitberger needle) plus an augmented consultation with placebo acupuncture plus a brief consulta-tion. The results indicate that the augmented consultation had statistically significant and clinically relevant benefits over the limited consultation for irritable bowel syndrome (IBS) [258].

One reason it is difficult to construct legitimate acupuncture placebos is that the *therapeutic theory* for acupuncture is not fully developed. In his detailed work on the placebo concept, Grünbaum insisted that what counts as a placebo is necessarily relative to a therapeutic theory [291,333]. Although it is beyond the scope of this work to discuss what Grünbaum meant by a therapeutic theory in great detail, it is clear that the therapeutic theory would include, among other things, a specification of the character-istic features of the experimental therapy. Since the characteristic features of acupuncture are difficult to identify and/or isolate, attempts to construct legitimate placebos for acupuncture seem misguided.

The fact that the characteristic features are difficult to identify and/ or isolate, emphatically does not imply nihilism about the possibility of evaluating acupuncture scientifically. Rather, it means that *until* we find a legitimate placebo, so-called "placebo"-controlled trials of acupuncture are unlikely to provide clinically meaningful results, and that we should con-sider other research designs, including "active" controlled trials, random-ized trials involving "no treatment" controls, and dose-response studies.

Of course, both "no treatment" controls and "active" controls suffer from problems of their own (see next chapter) and it would take us far afield to delve into any detail here. Yet the scope of the problems are certainly often exaggerated [334,335]. Certainly a "no treatment" controlled trial that reveals a dramatic effect would suffice as strong evidence.

7.6 Summary and solution to the problem with illegitimate placebo controls

Doctor (to patient): *First take the white pill with a glass of water, then take the yel-low pill with a glass of water, then take the red pill with a glass of water.*

Patient: *What on earth do I need so many pills for?*

Doctor: *You don't drink enough water.*

—ANONYMOUS JOKE

Placebo controls are best conceptualized as treatments in their own right that require complete descriptions in reports of trials. Unless the placebo controls are legitimate, they will lead to mistaken estimates of the experimental therapy's characteristic effects. I have shown that many placebo control therapies are not legitimate; moreover, because of practical limitations, it is likely that even our best attempts to construct legitimate placebo controls will fail. To make matters worse, different placebo controls, even if legitimate, can have very different effects, which creates confusion for patients, practitioners, and policy-makers when making a comparison across two separate 'placebo'-controlled trials.

To justify placebo control legitimacy, we should require that placebo controls be described in detail, and the features they are intended to control for must be specified so that we can judge whether the placebo control is legitimate. For example, instead of describing the control therapy in a trial of Prozac as a placebo control, investigators should provide a more precise description such as:

> A treatment intended to control for all the features of real Prozac save fluoxetine hydrochloride. The pill appears the same as a Prozac pill, but fluoxetine hydrochloride is replaced by lactose, and the pill is delivered in the same way as real Prozac, by masked investigators to masked participants. Tests at the end of the trial for the success of masking revealed that. . .

The treatment, once adequately described, should subsequently be referred to as the control treatment rather than the placebo. Indeed, there has recently been a call to abandon the term "placebo" altogether [302,303]. Although in the case of drug trials this may seem like overkill, the examples of olive oil placebos and unsuccessfully masked trials suggests that adequate description could be necessary more often than we think. In cases of non-drug treatments such as exercise therapy or acupuncture therapy, rather than the terms "sham exercise" or "sham acupuncture," which are highly ambiguous, a description such as "core flexibility exercises three times per week supervised by unmasked, qualified physiotherapists" would help prevent confusion.

CHAPTER 8

Questioning the methodological superiority of "placebo" over "active" controlled trials*

Let us examine the placebo somewhat more critically, however, since it and "double blind" have reached the status of fetishes in our thinking and literature. The Automatic Aura of Respectability, Infallibility, and Scientific Savoir-faire which they possess for many can be easily shown to be undeserved in certain circumstances.

—L. LASAGNA [249]

8.1 Epistemological foundations of the ethical debate over the use of placebo-controlled trials

Many have argued that only placebo-controlled trials (PCTs) and not "active" controlled trials (ACTs) provide reliable knowledge about therapeutic effects of medical treatments [334–338]. If it is the case that only PCTs provide the desired knowledge, then this would provide randomized trials with an additional benefit over observational studies since only the former can employ placebo controls.

---

*A slightly shorter version of this chapter was published in *American Journal of Bioethics* 2009;9:34–48.

The Philosophy of Evidence-Based Medicine, First Edition. Jeremy Howick.
© 2011 Jeremy Howick. Published 2011 by Blackwell Publishing Ltd.

However, the alleged methodological advantages of PCTs have been asserted more often than argued for. For instance, the revised Declaration of Helsinki states:

> a placebo controlled trial may be ethically acceptable even if proven therapy is available, under the following circumstances:
> – Where for compelling and scientifically sound methodological reasons *its use is necessary to determine the efficacy or safety of a prophylactic, diagnostic, or therapeutic method* [337].

Yet the authors are silent when it comes to specifying what the "compelling reasons" for requiring PCTs might be, let alone providing any arguments for why we should accept them. Likewise, Miller and Brody [338] devote one paragraph and cite only two sources [334,335] to justify their claim that ACTs suffer from methodological flaws. The International Conference on Harmonization (ICH) E10 document [336], produced and endorsed by the regulatory bodies of the USA, the European Union, and Japan lists the following alleged methodological flaws with ACTs.

1 ACTs do not always possess "assay sensitivity" whereas PCTs do.
2 ACTs do not provide a direct measure of absolute effect size whereas PCTs do.
3 ACTs require a larger sample size than PCTs.

But the document fails to defend the claims with sustained arguments. In this chapter I aim to address this oversight.

To anticipate, I will contend that outside cases where we have no established therapy, none of the arguments supporting the methodological superiority of PCTs are acceptable. Moreover, ACTs provide evidence that has a higher degree of patient relevance. What the average patient, clinician, and policy-maker needs to know is not whether a new treatment is better than a placebo, but whether the new therapy is better than what we already have. If I am correct that the arguments for the superiority of PCTs over ACTs are unsustainable, then it is rarely the case that the feature of being able to employ placebo controls confers an *additional* benefit to randomized trials over observational studies (however, the other benefits of randomized trials stand). Here, as elsewhere [1,47], ethics and epistemology are inseparable. Standards for ethical clinical practice from the Hippocratic Oath to more modern guidelines [339–341] require the clinician to provide the best available treatment. This moral duty would seem to require that the clinician avoid PCTs where there is an established therapy. Instead of PCTs, the ethical clinician should advocate ACTs that compare the new treatment with the best established treatment. On the other hand, if it were true that only PCTs provided reliable knowledge, then ACTs would be unethical. Poor-quality research cannot provide the desired knowledge, hence wastes scarce resources and exposes participants to unnecessary risks and burdens [342–346]. In short, the alleged methodological failings of ACTs seem to imply different ethical duties for clinicians and researchers. However, if I am correct that ACTs provide equally reliable knowledge, then the tension between clinical ethics and research ethics dissolves. The ethical duty of the clinician to avoid PCTs where established therapy is available is unchallenged by methodological considerations.

8.2 Problems with the assay sensitivity arguments against ACTs

Assay sensitivity is defined as the ability of a trial to distinguish differences between experimental and control therapies. However, there are two distinct versions of the definition, each leading to different arguments against ACTs. Temple and Ellenberg [334] define assay sensitivity as "The ability of a study to distinguish between active [non-placebo] and inactive [placebo] treatments." Others define assay sensitivity as "the ability to distinguish a more effective treatment from a less effective [placebo or not] treatment" [336,347]. The first assay sensitivity argument is that PCTs but not ACTs can distinguish between placebos and non-placebos, while the second is that PCTs but not ACTs can distinguish between more effective and less effective treatments. I will examine each argument in turn.

8.3 Problems with the first assay sensitivity argument against ACTs

The motivation for the first assay sensitivity argument is clear: most medical treatments used until at least the mid-19th century were either no better than placebo, or worse [348,349]. Even recently, careful investigation has uncovered that several widely used treatments were useless or harmful [24,209,350–356). History teaches us that we cannot always assume that our existing treatments are effective, as in "more effective than placebo." (NB We do not necessarily require a PCT to demonstrate effectiveness, i.e. superiority to placebo. To use a much-cited example, we do not need a placebo control to determine that parachute use is more effective than placebo, however "placebo" is defined [30].) If an experimental treatment demonstrates superiority to an established treatment that itself is less effective than placebo, we cannot conclude that the new agent is effective. In short, ACTs that employ useless or harmful treatments as controls will not possess assay sensitivity (of the first kind). Put differently, in order to claim an ACT possesses assay sensitivity we must assume that the control treatment was effective. Since there have been (and undoubtedly are) accepted treatments that are useless or harmful, not all ACTs will possess assay sensitivity.

PCTs, on the other hand, purportedly do not suffer from this problem. A "positive" result of a PCT, where the experimental treatment demonstrates superiority to placebo, appears to justify the inference to "effectiveness" without any external assumptions.

> A well-designed study that shows superiority of a treatment to a control . . . provides strong evidence of the [non-placebo] effectiveness of the new treatment, limited only by the statistical uncertainty of the result. No information external to the trial is needed to support the conclusion of effectiveness [335].

Or so it seems.

I will contend that the first assay sensitivity argument against ACTs is problematic in two ways. Firstly, PCTs can also lack assay sensitivity because actual placebo controls used in clinical trials can be either more or less effective than "real" placebos and, secondly, the argument is severely limited in scope.

8.3.1 Why PCTs suffer from assay sensitivity problems: actual placebo controls can be more, or less, effective than real placebos

We saw last chapter that many actual placebo controls used in trials are often illegitimate in the sense that they are either more, or less, effective than 'real' placebos. Besides the problem with illegitimate placebo controls, there is another reason why PCTs do not possess assay sensitivity (of the first kind): the effects of placebo controls vary widely. Moerman [299] found that while the effect of cimetidine for ulcers remained *relatively* constant across trials, the effectiveness of the placebos in the same trials ranged from 10 to 90% of the drug effect. An update of the review yielded more dramatic results, with the placebo effect ranging from 0 to 100% of the (again relatively constant) drug effect [357]. Another neuro-gastroenterological study of treatments for IBS found that the placebo response ranged from 16.0 to 71.4% of the (roughly constant) experimental treatment [358]. Although the reason for the substantial variation in placebo effects could be that the placebos in question were illegitimate, placebos could also have inherently variable effectiveness.

The variable placebo effects in trials with relatively constant experimental treatment effects present an assay sensitivity problem for PCTs. Are cimetidine and the IBS treatments effective? The answer depends on which relative response to placebo we assume to be "correct." But this places PCTs on the same footing as ACTs as far as assay sensitivity (of the first kind) is concerned. In order to assert that ACTs possess assay sensitivity, we must assume that the established treatment control was effective; in order to assert that PCTs possess assay sensitivity, we must assume that a particular placebo effect is "correct" (and legitimate).

We might object that it is unreasonable to generalize about the variability or illegitimacy of placebo response rate from a handful of studies. This objection can only be answered by further empirical work. Given the vital role of placebo controls in determining whether a treatment is deemed effective, it would be useful for methodologists to investigate the extent to which the effectiveness of placebo controls varies. Furthermore, it suffices for some PCTs to lack assay sensitivity in order for them to be as assay insensitive as ACTs. After all, as I shall now argue, most ACTs possess assay sensitivity.

8.3.2 The limited scope of the first assay sensitivity argument

ACTs will lack assay sensitivity when we have good reason to doubt the effectiveness of the established treatment control. But how often should we worry about the effects of our established therapies? In the early 1990s Smith [359] suggested that 80–90% of our treatments lacked a sound evidence base. However, these estimations may have equated "evidence" with "randomized evidence," which is a mistake. Many treatments, ranging from the Heimlich maneuver to tracheostomies, are undoubtedly effective yet they have not been tested in placebo-controlled randomized trials. More recent research indicates that between 76% (pediatric surgery) and 96% (anesthesia) of our current practice is based on compelling (randomized or non-randomized) evidence [360–362]. Since the majority of our current treatments are effective, the majority of ACTs will possess assay sensitivity. Moreover, in cases where we doubt the effectiveness of our current treatments we can simply require that a new treatment demonstrate superiority to the control. Then, provided that the existing treatment is not much *worse* than a placebo, the ACT will possess assay sensitivity. As we shall soon see, new treatments are often, and in my view unjustifiably, required to demonstrate rough equivalence (or "non-inferiority") to established treatments rather than superiority.

Although Temple and Ellenberg acknowledge that the assay sensitivity argument is limited in scope, they might object that the problem with

ACTs is more severe than I have indicated. They argue (rather oddly) that a treatment can be undoubtedly effective yet fail to demonstrate this effectiveness reliably: "the effectiveness of [some] drugs that sometimes (or even often) fail to be proven superior to 'placebo' is not in doubt" [334]. The supposed problem is allegedly neither with trial size nor quality, but rather with the failure of the trial to reveal the effects of the experimental treatment for some unknown reason: "In each case . . . the problem [of assay sensitivity] is not identifiable a priori by examining the study; it is recognized only by the observed failure of the trial to distinguish the drug and placebo treatments" [334].

If Temple and Ellenberg are correct, then the first assay sensitivity argument applies *somewhat* more widely than I have indicated. Temple and Ellenberg mention 11 classes of treatments that have assay sensitivity problems, provide some evidence for four of these classes, and only discuss SSRIs in any detail. We could grant that there are treatments with assay sensitivity problems and still assert that the first assay sensitivity argument was limited in scope.

A deeper problem, however, is that the idea of treatments with assay sensitivity problems is hard to swallow. Indeed, properly speaking treatments *cannot* have assay sensitivity problems because assay sensitivity is a property of trials rather than treatments. What Temple and Ellenberg mean is that if treatments do not demonstrate their effects reliably, then ACTs using these treatments as controls can (allegedly) be at risk from assay insensitivity. But the way we determine that a treatment has an effect is by testing it in well-controlled trials. If trials fail to detect effects, then there is good reason to doubt whether the effect exists. To blame a trial for not detecting the effects begs the question.

Temple and Ellenberg might respond with a probabilistic argument for accepting that there are treatments with assay sensitivity problems [334]:

> even if a drug is statistically significantly superior to placebo in only 50% of well-designed and well-conducted studies, that proportion will still be vastly greater than the small fraction that would be expected to occur by chance if the drugs were ineffective.

However, the probabilistic argument is unacceptable for two reasons. First, it ignores the possibility of systematic bias and second it fails to consider that the treatment appeared harmful in the other 50% of trials. Publication bias [363], funding source bias [364], and bias introduced by underdiagnosed methodological problems such as failure to keep a trial successfully masked [266,267] will tend to exaggerate the size of the apparent experimental treatment effect. In cases where the absolute effect size of the treatment is small (as is the case for SSRIs), ruling out these biases could well reduce the number of "positive" studies to well within what we would expect by chance alone (see conclusion). Furthermore, a treatment that is effective in 50% of trials could be harmful in the remaining 50%. Systematic reviews (which Temple and Ellenberg fail to discuss) would be a good way to con-firm claims that treatments with assay sensitivity problems have overall positive effects. In fact systematic reviews of SSRIs – Temple and Ellenberg's paradigmatic example of drugs with assay sensitivity problems – are ambiguous. While the Cochrane review concludes that there are small differences between active placebo and SSRIs [192], other systematic reviews failed to detect statistically significant benefits of SSRIs over placebo [25–28,365].

I am not pronouncing on the debate over the antidepressant effects of SSRIs. Rather, I am disputing the claim that SSRIs have such indubitable effects that any trial failing to detect such effects, no matter how well con-trolled or large, must be flawed. A plausible alternative explanation for the failure to demonstrate effects in large and well-controlled trials is that the *treatments are ineffective*.

Most importantly, the problem with control treatments that might have assay sensitivity problems presents a worry for PCTs as much as ACTs. Imagine a new SSRI was developed that, like other SSRIs, had assay sensi-tivity problems. If the first few trials in which the new SSRI were tested did not possess assay sensitivity (and the drug failed to demonstrate superior-ity to placebo), it would be dropped before its supposedly undoubted effec-tiveness was detected. Thus, the potential existence of drugs with assay sensitivity problems does not provide us with any reason to prefer PCTs.

The scope of the first assay sensitivity argument is further limited if we require that new agents demonstrate *superiority* to the control treat-ments. Even if an established treatment is ineffective (but is no worse than placebo) or has assay sensitivity problems, provided it demonstrated superiority to its predecessor, we could conclude that the new agent is more effective than a placebo. In practice, however, many new agents are not required to demonstrate superiority but rather (rough) equivalence in *non-inferiority* trials.

Briefly (more will follow), a "non-inferiority" trial is designed to detect whether the experimental intervention is at least of equal (to within some margin of equivalence) effectiveness to the control treatment (Figure 8.1). 'Superiority' trials, on the other hand, are designed to detect whether the experimental treatment is more effective than the control.

Non-inferiority trials are justified in some cases. For example, the extra-cranial/intracranial anastomosis (EC/IC) Bypass Study Group contrasted

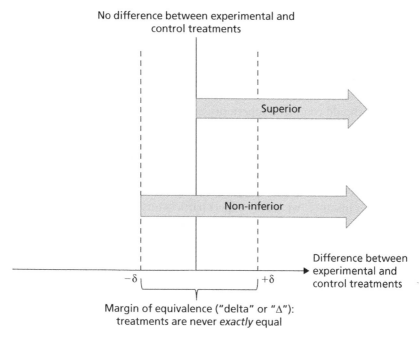

Figure 8.1 The difference between superiority and non-inferiority.

no treatment with surgery (superficial temporal artery–middle cerebral artery anastomosis) for patients with a high risk of stroke [366]. A non-inferiority test revealed that doing nothing was not worse (to within 3%) than surgery. In this case, and a few others [367], non-inferiority tests have led to the *rejection* of relatively risky, invasive, and expensive procedures. More recently, however, non-inferiority trials have justified the adoption of many treatments that are no better than our existing treatments, and usually far more expensive [368].

The justification for non-inferiority trials is that treatments can allegedly represent a real advance without offering superiority on the primary out-come. More specifically [369,370]:

1 the new treatment might have fewer side-effects;
2 the new treatment could be cheaper or less invasive;
3 the new treatment may be necessary in case people develop resistance to existing therapies.

Although the rationale for non-inferiority trials appears sensible, I will argue that non-inferiority trials rarely help us discover whether a new treatment has one of these advantages.

Comparisons of side-effects are often made carelessly. Existing treatments have usually been around for longer, so there will be more extensive data about their side-effects. Certainly rare and long-term side-effects of the new treatment will be relatively under-studied. Thus comparisons between the side-effects of newer and older treatments are often unbalanced. In addition, if the new treatment has a better side-effect profile, then we should conduct a superiority test of the relevant side-effects. It is, of course, possible to run a superiority test for the side-effects of interest and a non-inferiority test for the main outcome simultaneously.

If the new treatment is supposed to be more tolerable because it is less invasive or more convenient – say it involves one daily dose instead of two – then the benefits of the new regimen should result in a superior outcome [371]. For instance, we would expect participants taking one dose per day to adhere better to the regimen. The superior adherence should translate to better outcomes. If not, then it is unclear whether the apparent improved convenience is of any value. At least in principle, apparently less convenient or more invasive regimens could improve the primary outcome, perhaps by enhancing the placebo response.

Next, even if we allow *some* non-inferior treatments in case people develop resistance to our existing therapies or an unexpected side-effect is discovered, it does not follow that we need dozens of similar therapies. Yet dozens of roughly equivalent treatments is just what indiscriminate use of non-inferiority trials encourages. For instance, there are currently over six SSRI antidepressants, and numerous other pharmaceutical antidepressants (tricyclics, monoamine oxidase inhibitors, serotonin/norepinephrine reuptake inhibitors, norepinephrine and specific serotonergic antidepressants, norepinephrine reuptake inhibitors, and norepinephrine–dopamine reuptake inhibitors). In addition, there are many non-pharmaceutical treatments used to treat depression, including St John's Wort, cognitive behavior therapy, exercise, and self-help. None of these treatments have demonstrated consistent superiority to others in trials, although the administration of some (e.g. exercise) is admittedly very different from others. Even if it were useful to have a few of these treatments available in case one of them suddenly turned out to be harmful or because patients somehow developed resistance, it is difficult to justify so many.

Finally, non-inferiority trials present an ethical problem for the clinician. If the experimental treatment is *at best* roughly equal, but could be worse, then the best available therapy is probably the existing one. It is unclear whether the ethical clinician should allow her patient to risk receiving an inferior treatment.

In brief, non-inferiority trials cannot be deemed worthwhile without special justification. Accordingly, institutional review boards (IRBs) should investigate requests to approve non-inferiority trials more carefully. Market constraints might make it difficult in practice to officially restrict the number of non-inferior treatments, but it does not follow that non-inferiority trials are morally justified.

To recap what has been argued thus far, PCTs suffer from assay sensitivity problems much like ACTs because placebo controls can be illegitimate, and their effectiveness varies widely. In addition, the scope of the first assay sensitivity argument is limited to non-inferiority ACTs where we have reason to doubt the effects of the control treatment, and non-inferiority trials are rarely justified.

Before considering the second assay sensitivity argument, I will say a few words about hybrid trial designs that involve both active and placebo controls. Some trials, for example, have three groups: experimental, existing treatment, and placebo. One might think that three-armed trials can be used to compare the experimental treatment with an existing therapy *and* test whether the trial possessed assay sensitivity. However, the three-armed solution remains problematic for the clinician who seems morally compelled to use the best available treatment. Besides, the three-armed solution is only an improvement over regular ACTs if we believe that adding the placebo group will make the trial assay sensitive, which the above (and subsequent) discussion suggests is not the case.

Another hybrid trial design that employs both placebo and active controls is the placebo-controlled add-on trial. Here, all patients in the trial receive the best existing therapy. Then, some receive the new agent *in addition* (i.e. an "add-on") to the existing therapy, while others receive a placebo in addition to the existing therapy [372]. This design overcomes the ethical objections to conventional placebo-controlled trials, and is useful for discovering whether a new therapy would be a good adjunct to existing therapy. It is also useful for discovering whether a new therapy might benefit those who did not respond to existing therapy. However, as far as the non-responders to existing therapy are concerned, there is no *established* existing therapy, and a superiority ACT might be easier to conduct. Other problems with this design include the fact that it would not tell us which single therapy is generally more beneficial in cases where multiple treatments are unnecessary or unfeasible, and it would not be appropriate if the new and established agents interacted (see section 8.5).

Yet a another trial design that employs both placebo and active controls is the "double-dummy" design where patients receive both a placebo and an active treatment. This technique is particularly useful when we wish to compare two outwardly distinguishable therapies in double-masked conditions. For example, if we wish to compare injections and tablets, we could give one group "active" injections and "placebo" tablets, and the other group "placebo" injections and "active" tablets. While this design involves placebos, it is not a PCT in the sense described above because the purpose of the trial is to compare two active treatments rather than measure whether a new agent is superior to placebo.

8.4 The second assay sensitivity argument

Recall that the term "assay sensitivity" is also defined as the ability of a trial to distinguish between more effective and less effective (placebo or not) treatments. The second assay sensitivity argument is then that PCTs but not ACTs are able to detect differences between experimental and control treatments. Since the structure of superiority ACTs and superiority PCTs is identical as far as detecting differences are concerned, this argument applies exclusively to non-inferiority ACTs. Hence the second assay sensitivity argument is also limited in scope because it only applies to often unjustified non-inferiority ACTs.

Moreover, whereas the purpose of non-inferiority trials is not to detect differences, they are as *capable* as superiority trials of detecting differences. Although some discussion of classical statistics is necessary to understand why I believe this argument fails, I will keep the current discussion intuitive and as non-technical as possible. The reader is referred to the Appendix and other sources for a more detailed treatment [189,334,347,370,373–376).

Both superiority and non-inferiority can be tested using confidence intervals. A confidence interval represents a range within which the mean difference between experimental and control treatments is likely to lie (Figure 8.2). If the entire confidence interval lies to the right of the line representing no difference (the solid vertical line in Figure 8.2), we can conclude (in a probabilistic sense) that the experimental treatment is superior. If the entire confidence interval lies to the right of the lower bound of the equivalence margin ($-\delta$ in Figure 8.2), we can conclude (again in a probabilistic sense) non-inferiority. It is true that a positive result of a non-inferiority trial does not provide evidence of a difference: a treatment could be non-inferior and also roughly equal (the confidence interval could lie within the equivalence margin bound by $-\delta$ and $+\delta$ in Figure 8.2). It is also true that the purpose of a non-inferiority trial is not to detect a difference – we would be happy if the experimental treatment were roughly equal. It does not follow, however, that a non-inferiority trial *cannot* detect a difference. Even if the purpose of the trial is to detect non-inferiority, if we find that the confidence interval lies entirely to either side of the line representing no difference, then the trial will have provided evidence that a treatment difference exists.

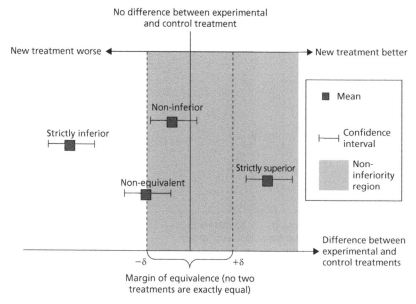

Figure 8.2 The difference between superiority and non-inferiority trials using confidence intervals.

Hence it is trivially false that non-inferiority ACTs are less capable of detecting differences than PCTs.

I will now examine the argument that PCTs (but not ACTs) provide a measure of absolute effect size.

8.5 Challenging the view that PCTs provide a measure of absolute effect size

It is often alleged that PCTs are superior to ACTs on the grounds that only the former provide a measure of absolute effect size:

> The placebo-controlled trial measures the total pharmacologically mediated effect of treatment. In contrast an active controlled trial . . . measures the effect relative to another treatment. . . . The *absolute* effect size information is valuable [my emphasis] [336].

I will argue that we must make two unwarranted assumptions in order to assert that PCTs provide a measure of absolute effect size. The first, *additivity*, is that the placebo and non-placebo components of a treatment add

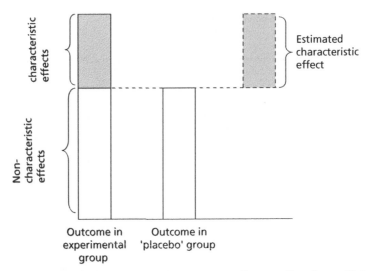

Figure 8.3 How the absolute measure of characteristic effects are allegedly provided by PCTs.

(like vectors) rather than interact (like compounds in a chemical reaction). The second assumption is that placebo controls are legitimate.

Additivity is the assumption that the various treatment factors combine like vectors rather than chemicals in a reaction. For example, we can dissect a force propelling a billiard ball in a northeasterly direction into its northward and eastward components. Since the component forces act independently we can deduce the resultant force if we know the magnitude and direction of its components [170]. If additivity held in PCTs, then if we knew the *combined* effect of the characteristic and non-characteristic features (measured in the experimental group), and we also knew the effect of the non-characteristic features (measured in the placebo group), then we could deduce the absolute effect of the characteristic features (Figure 8.3).

However, it is unclear why we should assume that the characteristic and non-characteristic treatment features add rather than interact. Certainly additivity does not usually apply to the combination of chemical, biological, or even non-mechanical physical causes. For example, the combination of hydrogen and oxygen produces water, which does not retain the properties of either hydrogen or oxygen [170]. In fact there is some evidence to support the view that placebo and non-placebo components of a treatment process interact rather than add.

Evidence for interactions between characteristic and non-characteristic features is sparse. Yet the paucity of evidence must not be taken as evidence that interactions are rare. Aside from a few interesting papers [377–379], the assumption of additivity has been largely ignored. It would be helpful for methodologists to investigate the issue further. Until the assumption has been examined more carefully, it is difficult to draw conclusions about the prevalence of interactions. With that in mind, the modest intent of this section is to show that additivity cannot be taken for granted.

In the studies cited earlier about the variable effects of placebos for cimetidine and IBS-therapy placebos, the characteristic features did not add to the non-characteristic features. Rather, they interacted in such a way that the characteristic benefit tapered off as the strength of the placebo (non-characteristic) features increased. If the characteristic and non-characteristic components were additive, changing the effects of non-characteristic features would not change the effect of the characteristic features (changing the magnitude of the eastward force on a billiard ball will not affect its northward motion).

In other cases, the magnitude of the non-characteristic features has been manipulated experimentally and the resulting characteristic effectiveness changed. For instance, Hughes *et al.* [380] investigated the effects of nicotine gum for smoking cessation. The trial involved 77 participants who provided their informed consent to have a 50/50 chance of receiving nicotine or placebo gum, and that they might or might not be told the contents of their gum. They were *not* told that they could be deceived. (It is unlikely that IRBs would approve such a trial to be conducted today.) The participants were then assigned to one of six groups (Table 8.1). Two groups (1 and 2) were told they would receive placebo (and thus had low expectations regarding recovery), two (3 and 4) were told they would receive real nicotine gum (and thus had higher expectations regarding recovery), while the remaining two groups (5 and 6) were delivered either placebo or nicotine gum under double-masked conditions (and thus had 'medium' expectations regarding recovery). Only one group from each pair (1, 3, 5) was

Table 8.1 The extended balanced placebo design used in the study of the effects of nicotine gum (Hughes *et al.* [380])

Told	Received	
	Treatment	No treatment
Treatment	1	2
No treatment	3	4
Neither (treatment delivered in double-masked conditions)	5	6

actually given nicotine gum; the other was given placebo. All participants, especially those in the two groups told they were given a placebo, were encouraged to use the gum whenever the urge to smoke occurred.

The outcome measures were proportion of participants who smoked no cigarettes during the week, proportion who smoked on fewer than 2 days per week, number of days smoked per week, and number of cigarettes smoked per week. These were calculated based on assessments measured 1 and 2 weeks after participants attempted to quit, and were measured in three ways. First, the participants self-reported how many cigarettes they smoked. Second, a designated observer (usually a spouse) reported the participant's smoking habits during the week. Third, a breath sample of carbon monoxide was taken to verify claims of complete abstinence.

The characteristic benefit of real nicotine gum was not a constant that added to the benefit of the varying non-characteristic features. Rather, the characteristic effects tapered off as the strength of expectations increased (Figure 8.4). The statistical evidence for interactions between instructions and the overall outcome was significant ($P = 0.01$).

Several other studies employing similar designs also indicate that additivity does not hold. Analgesic response [381], amphetamine effects [382], and subjective feelings of intoxication [383] have all been shown to decrease as the strength of expectations increases. One study even

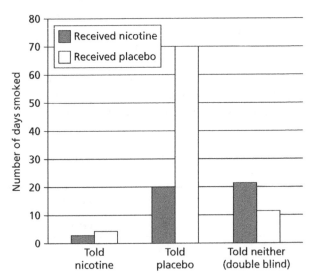

Figure 8.4 Smoking behavior by instruction and drug group. The results are cumulative across the 2 weeks where assessments were made. Based on Hughes *et al.* [380].

indicates that the increased "strength" of non-characteristic features of treatment with naloxone can change the apparent benefit of the characteristic features from positive to negative [381].

Interestingly, these studies all indicate that trial findings, at least for these ailments, may not apply to routine practice where expectations are often quite different. The nicotine gum trial, for instance, suggests that in routine practice, where presumably expectations are high, there would not be any characteristic benefit of the gum. Since expectations in ACTs are, on average, closer to expectations in routine practice expectations than in PCTs, the external validity of ACTs is higher than in PCTs.

It is also possible for non-characteristic and characteristic features to combine synergistically. For example, Freud argued that charging a hefty fee might act as a catalyst for what are commonly thought of as the characteristic features of Freudian psychoanalysis [291,384].

We need not resort to mysterious explanations to account for interactions. Many ailments can only be relieved by so much. If the expectations alone produce this maximum effect (or something close to it), then there will be little room for drug-induced improvement. Once a headache is completely relieved, taking another pill will not relieve it further. The mechanism that accounts for a maximum drug response is often understood [385]. To oversimplify, the maximum response is often related to the maximum number of receptors that cells have for the drug to attach to. Once all the receptors are occupied, there is no further room for improvement. If expectations and beliefs spur the body to produce an agent that occupies these receptors, then the drug will not have its otherwise significant effect. Synergistic interactions can also be explained. There is evidence that placebos for pain increase the levels of endogenous opioids [292,386]. The increased opioid level could stimulate interaction with the characteristic features to increase the effects by interacting synergistically with the active treatment.

These examples suffice to show that additivity cannot be taken for granted. Even where additivity might hold, however, another assumption must be made to support the claim that PCTs provide a measure of absolute effect size: the performance of the placebo controls must be legitimate and perform consistently.

Unless placebo controls are legitimate, they do not provide a baseline against which the characteristic effects (absolute or not) of the treatment can be measured. But we saw in the last chapter that placebo controls are not always legitimate. Likewise, the Moerman and Patel studies indicate that the wide variability of placebo control treatments (legitimate or not) can determine how effective an experimental treatment appears. It would indeed be a strange definition of absolute effect size that was compatible with the effect size changing drastically from study to study.

In brief, the assumptions (i) that the characteristic and non-characteristic treatment features add rather than interact, and (ii) that the placebo controls are legitimate are rarely, if ever, jointly justified. As a result, the claim that PCTs provide an absolute measure of effect size cannot be maintained.

8.6 Questioning the claim that PCTs require smaller sample sizes

A final alleged benefit of PCTs is that they require smaller sample sizes than ACTs [336]. It is an ethical requirement to use the smallest possible sample size since smaller trials are cheaper and expose fewer participants to risk. However, it is unclear that the sample size issue in particular and practical considerations in general weigh in on the side of PCTs.

For one, only non-inferiority ACTs allegedly require a larger sample size than PCTs. Then, the supposed reason why PCTs require a smaller sample size is that the equivalence margin (see Figure 8.1) is often much smaller than the treatment difference that a PCT is designed to detect. Yet if a PCT is designed to detect a difference which is the same size as the equivalence margin, then it will require an equally large sample size.

Besides, there are several practical considerations that reduce the force of the claim that PCTs are preferable because they require a smaller sample size even if it were true. For one, potential participants may be more likely to consent to a trial where they are certain to receive an active treatment than they would be if they might get a placebo. Similarly, PCTs might face a more acute threat from the fact that participants seem to be quite good at detecting which group they are in despite efforts to keep the trial blind [266,267]. A participant in a PCT who guesses she is taking the placebo might well drop out or covertly seek treatment outside the trial. On the other hand, a participant in an ACT who guesses he is in the control group is already (supposedly) taking the best available treatment, and will have less incentive to drop out or seek outside treatment.

Next, a further study is required in order to apply the results of a PCT. In order to make an informed choice about whether to use the new treatment, the patient, practitioner, or policy-maker must know how the new treatment compares with the best existing treatments rather than how it compares with placebo. This information would have to be obtained from an additional ACT, or an indirect comparative study. The human and financial burden of the additional study would have to be added to the cost of the PCT before asserting that PCTs are preferable because they require fewer participants than ACTs. In reality, of course, the further studies are rarely done. If not, then we must take into account the risk of doing harm or of allocating scarce resources to an inferior treatment when assessing the relative practical benefits of PCTs.

Lastly, what the average patient, practitioner, and policy-maker needs to know in order to decide to use a new treatment is how it compares with the best existing treatment, not how it compares with placebo. In short, the alleged practical advantages of PCTs have been exaggerated, while the practical disadvantages of PCTs have been overlooked.

8.7 Conclusion: a reassessment of the relative methodological quality of PCTs

Even if taken on their own terms, both assay sensitivity arguments are strictly limited in scope to non-inferiority ACTs where the control treatment is ineffective or has assay sensitivity problems. More fundamentally, neither assay sensitivity argument is acceptable. The first fails because PCTs sometimes lack assay sensitivity and ACTs often possess it. The second is based on a conflation of the difference between the purpose and properties of non-inferiority trials. The argument that PCTs provide a measure of the absolute effect of the characteristic features of the experimental treatment relies on rarely warranted assumptions that placebo controls are legitimate and that characteristic and non-characteristic treatment features add rather than interact. Lastly, practical considerations, including sample size, often support ACTs rather than PCTs. Judged as arguments that ACTs are methodologically superior to PCTs, all three arguments must be judged as failures. Claims [334–338] about the methodological superiority of PCTs over ACTs are therefore unjustified.

The results of this chapter dissolves the apparent tension between clinical and research ethics as far as the use of placebo controls is concerned. The ethical duty of the clinician to provide the best care (and avoid PCTs) when there is an established treatment available stands unchallenged by the moral duties of the clinical researcher to use the best method. The Declaration of Helsinki should retract the statement that PCTs can be justified on methodological grounds (where there is an available established therapy) and IRBs should dismiss claims that PCTs are methodologically superior to ACTs as grounds to approve PCTs where standard therapy is available.

Moreover, the conclusions of this chapter imply that the practically unique feature of being able to employ placebo controls does not confer randomized trials with an additional potential benefit over observational studies. However, the other advantages of randomized trials listed in the previous chapters stand.

Appendix: more detailed explanation of why the second assay sensitivity argument fails

In classical hypothesis testing, hypotheses are not confirmed, but they can be rejected (in a probabilistic sense). We therefore attempt to reject the "null hypothesis" that represents the *opposite* of what we would like to establish. If we succeed, this is generally taken to support the alternative hypothesis. In a one-tailed superiority PCT, the null hypothesis is that there is no difference between experimental treatment and placebo, or that the experimental treatment is less effective than placebo. The alternative hypothesis will be that the experimental treatment is superior to the placebo (Figure 8.5).

A non-inferiority trial is designed to determine whether the experimental treatment is at least (roughly) equal in effectiveness to the control treatment. Therefore, we seek to rule out the null hypothesis that the experimental treatment is less effective by at least some minimum amount than the control treatment. The alternative hypothesis in a non-inferiority

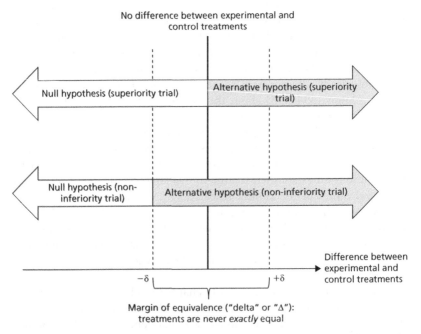

Figure 8.5 Illustration of null and alternative hypotheses in one-tailed superiority and one-tailed non-inferiority trials.

Table 8.2 The difference between type I and type II errors for superiority (PCT) and non-inferiority (ACT) trials

	Evidence for difference	
	Superiority (PCT)	Non-inferiority (ACT)
Low type I error rate (false positive)	Yes*	No
Low type II error (false negative)	No	Yes

*"Yes" means that there is evidence of a difference; "No" means that there is no evidence for difference. For example, a superiority trial with a low type I error rate provides good evidence for a difference.

trial is that the experimental treatment is of equal or greater effectiveness (Figure 8.5).

Whether a trial is good at detecting differences depends on how high the risk of type I and type II errors are. A type I error, or "false positive," is the error of rejecting a true null hypothesis (and accepting a false alternative hypothesis). A type II error, or "false negative," is the mistake of failing to reject a false null hypothesis (and not accepting a true alternative hypothesis). In a superiority trial, a type I error is the mistake of accepting a positive difference when there is none, while a type II error is the mistake of accepting no difference or inferiority when the experimental treatment is superior. A type I error in a non-inferiority trial is the mistake of accepting rough equality or superiority when the experimental treatment is strictly inferior, while a type II error is the mistake of accepting strict inferiority when the experimental treatment is roughly equal or superior.

Both type I and type II errors can be controlled for and specified in advance of a trial. To sensitize a superiority trial to differences, we reduce the type I error rate. To sensitize a non-inferiority trial to differences we must reduce the type II error rate (Table 8.2).

With this in mind, it is straightforward to show that non-inferiority trials are as good (or bad) at detecting differences as superiority trials. The discussion below follows Anderson [387]. Anderson postulates four conditions required to assume assay sensitivity. Using D to denote "difference between intervention and control group" and T to denote "trial," the conditions for asserting assay sensitivity (of the second kind) are

1 D
2 T indicates D
3 D → (T indicates D)
4 not-D → not (T indicates D).

The first condition tells us that, ontologically speaking, there is a difference between the interventions being compared. The second tells us that the trial indicated a difference. The third tells us that the trial would indicate a difference if there were one. The fourth tells us that if there is no difference, then the trial will not indicate a difference. In the real world, of course, the modality of the conditionals in (3) and (4) is not necessity – actual trials deal in probability.

The four conditions for assay sensitivity will be satisfied in a superiority trial when:

1 there is a difference (the experimental treatment is superior to placebo)
2 the trial indicates a difference (there is a "positive" result)
3 the type II error rate is sufficiently low (the trial did not wrongly suggest no difference)
4 the type I error rate is sufficiently low (the trial did not wrongly indicate a difference).

In a non-inferiority trial, the four conditions for affirming assay sensitivity will be satisfied when

1 there is a difference (the experimental treatment is superior to placebo)
2 the trial indicates a difference (there is a "positive" result)
3 the type I error rate is sufficiently low
4 the type II error rate is sufficiently low.

As long as we are able to reduce both the type I and type II error rates sufficiently, *both* superiority and non-inferiority trials can be made equally assay sensitive. Anderson concludes, and he is surely correct, that "Contrary to the assay sensitivity argument, there is not an absolute difference between PCTs and ACTs with respect to . . . the assay sensitivity assumption" [387].

PART III

Examining the paradox that traditional roles for mechanistic reasoning and expert judgment have been up-ended by EBM

CHAPTER 9

Transition to Part III

9.1 Summary of Part II

Randomized trials rule out self-selection bias and allocation bias while observational studies do not. Hence, all other things being equal, it appears as though randomized trials provide better evidence than observational studies. However, this view leads to the paradox of effectiveness whereby our most effective therapies do not appear to be supported by best evidence. The paradox can be resolved by replacing the categorical ranking of randomized trials above observational studies with the requirement that in order to accept that a treatment has clinically relevant effects, the treatment must demonstrate an effect that outweighs the combined effect of plausible confounders. The flip side of this rule is that randomized trials that do not demonstrate a sufficiently large effect should be questioned (see Figure 5.1). Moreover, rather than being arranged in a hierarchy, different (sufficiently high-quality) types of evidence can provide mutual support for a hypothesis that a medical intervention produced its clinically relevant benefits.

Randomized trials have two other potential benefits over observational studies: they can employ double masking and placebo controls. *Successful* double masking rules out the potentially confounding influence of participant and caregiver beliefs and therefore should be regarded as a methodological virtue. However, the view that double-masked trials always provide stronger evidence leads to the Philip's paradox that our most effective treatments are unsupportable by best evidence. The paradox can be resolved by noting that the *potentially* confounding factors ruled out by double masking

The Philosophy of Evidence-Based Medicine, First Edition. Jeremy Howick.
© 2011 Jeremy Howick. Published 2011 by Blackwell Publishing Ltd.

are not *actual* confounders when the factors are related to the positive effects of the experimental treatment on the target disorder. The arguments that PCTs provide more reliable knowledge are unacceptable unless there is no established therapy. In fact, the term "placebo" is ambiguous: to avoid the ambiguity placebos are best conceptualized as treatments in their own right that deserve detailed description. Hence, the fact that randomized trials but not observational studies are able to employ double masking and placebo controls only provides randomized trials with an actual advantage when effect sizes are relatively modest and when there is no established therapy.

9.2 Introduction to Part III

The main aim of Part III will be to evaluate the EBM claim that mechanistic reasoning and expert judgment deserve their position below comparative clinical studies in the EBM hierarchy of evidence. I will argue that while the EBM position is acceptable on the whole, mechanistic reasoning can provide strong evidence in certain well-defined cases. Rather than being ranked below comparative clinical studies in a hierarchy, I mechanistic reasoning of sufficiently high quality should be weighed alongside evidence from comparative clinical studies. Meanwhile, expert judgment, while perhaps unimportant as *evidence*, plays several other roles that deserve more discussion in the EBM literature.

To avoid misunderstanding, I should emphasize from the outset that the EBM movement has always recognized the importance of the non-evidential roles of mechanistic reasoning and expert judgment [12]. EBM proponents claim that mechanistic reasoning is important for generalizing results of clinical trials to more general populations, and that expert judgment is important for integrating best evidence with patient values and circumstances. While these other roles are equally important as far as clinical decision-making is concerned, they are not, properly speaking, to do with justifying claims that medical treatments have their putative effects.

A secondary aim of Part III will be to address an unresolved issue from Part II, namely applying evidence to actual clinical decisions. Even the best systematic review of randomized trials will not always guide us to the right course of action for an individual in routine practice for two reasons. First, although results from randomized trials may apply to target populations more often than has been supposed [235–237], the problem with external validity is very real. This problem is confounded by the uncertainty inherent to all science and medicine in particular. Any study, no matter how well controlled, could have been confounded in some way, and moreover medical treatments generally work in a probabilistic sense.

In Part III of this book, we will see that mechanistic reasoning [52,56] and expert judgment [64] are often touted as solutions to the problems. In Chapter 10 I will argue that EBM proponents have exaggerated the importance of mechanistic reasoning for generalizing the results of a study, and in Chapter 11 I will review a body of largely ignored literature suggesting that expert judges are not good at predicting how individuals in routine practice will respond to therapies.

Second – and many have overlooked this point – no particular course of action follows from determining whether a medical intervention works. This is related to the error well known to philosophers of deriving an 'ought' from an 'is' [388]. Other factors, including patient circumstances and values, must be considered before prescribing a treatment. To use an example I will discuss in more detail in Chapter 11, it is no use telling an Olympic athlete about to row in the final that the best treatment is 3 days of bed rest if there is a second most effective therapy that will allow him to compete. With that in mind, in Chapter 11 I will contend that expert judgment is required to integrate best evidence with patient values and circumstances.

CHAPTER 10

A qualified defence of the EBM stance on mechanistic reasoning

...it is necessary to destroy completely the vain, little and, as it were, apish imitations of the world, which have been formed in various systems of philosophy by men's fancies.

—Francis Bacon [389]

10.1 A tension between proponents of mechanistic reasoning and EBM views

Mechanisms are all the rage in current philosophical work on causality [390–402), where relatively strong ontological claims are made on their behalf. Mechanisms are allegedly responsible for generating causal regularities – if not all causal regularities, at least a good number of causal regularities of central interest in science. Expressing this view quite clearly, Glennan states "a mechanical theory of causation suggests that two events are causally connected when and only when there is a mechanism connecting them" [399]. Much of the detailed work centres on the life sciences, where hosts of mechanisms are described and defended as the source of causal regularities. Here are just a couple of examples to give a sense of what these claims amount to. In the article that was a catalyst for the recent flurry of work on mechanisms, Machamer *et al.* [401] study the mechanism of protein synthesis, which they say gives rise to the association between RNA and protein; William Bechtel and Adele Abrahamsen

---

The Philosophy of Evidence-Based Medicine, First Edition. Jeremy Howick.

[390] study the mechanism for a metabolic system which they claim gives rise to the association between phosphoenolpyruvate and acetyl-CoA; and Stuart Glennan [400] discusses the genetic mechanism for producing offspring with blue eyes.

Besides underwriting causal phenomena, philosophers of science have argued that mechanisms are required for understanding [401], explanation [390,392], generalizing causal hypotheses [37,56], analyzing reasoning in discovery [390], unification [395], and for solving Hume's problem [399]. More recently, the work on mechanisms has expanded into the social sciences [233] and medicine [403].

If mechanisms play such essential roles, especially in underwriting causal regularities in the life sciences, it seems reasonable to expect that evidence about the nature, structure, and functioning of mechanisms should play a central role in supporting claims about the effectiveness of medical interventions since these are just a special subset of causal regularity claims: causal regularity claims with medical interventions as inputs and change in patient relevant outcomes as outputs. Indeed, Russo and Williamson insist on just this. Causal regularities are not well supported, they maintain, until good evidence is available about the mechanisms that give rise to them. In their words, "To establish causal claims, scientists need the mutual support of mechanisms and dependencies" [403]. Gillies [404] has written in support of Russo and Williamson's thesis but has subsequently (in conversation) retracted his support.

In stark contrast with Russo and Williamson's view, we have seen that EBM proponents do not rate mechanistic evidence at all highly. While they do not attack the potential *ontological* importance of mechanisms, mechanistic evidence does not even appear on some dominant evidence-ranking schemes [19]. In short, far from mechanistic evidence being central in the support of effectiveness claims, it is hardly to be counted evidence at all. Is this reasonable?

This chapter will explore a number of problems that beset the use of mechanistic evidence to support claims about the effects of medical interventions. The problems I raise will not depend on attacking the fundamental ontological issue – are these causal regularities underwritten for the most part by mechanisms – rather I shall stay neutral on this. Instead I shall raise problems with the potential evidential role of mechanisms. However, my overall conclusion will not be in support of the EBM view that mechanistic evidence is not evidence at all. Rather, I shall argue that where problems with our relevant knowledge of mechanisms can be overcome (and I will demonstrate with examples that sometimes they can), mechanistic reasoning can and should be used to support claims that medical interventions have their putative patient-relevant effects. I will conclude with some remarks about the potential usefulness of mechanisms for generalizing the results of clinical trials.

10.2 Clarifying the terminology: comparative clinical studies, mechanisms, and mechanistic reasoning

Mechanistic reasoning is best understood when contrasted with what the EBM movement believe provides the strongest evidential support, namely comparative clinical studies. Comparative clinical studies have been referred to as Mill's methods [170], the "numerical" method [8], the "statistical" method [9], and "difference-making" evidence [403]. The main idea behind these methods is the same. Recall from chapter 2 that in comparative clinical studies, some ("experimental") groups take the experimental intervention (I) while other ("control") groups do not. Then, outcomes (O) in the experimental and control groups are compared. If the outcome rates differ, the study counts as evidence that the intervention had an effect (that I caused O) (Figure 10.1).

A famous example of a comparative clinical study is the Cardiac Arrhythmia Suppression Trial (CAST), which began in 1987. The trial was designed to test whether antiarrhythmic drugs would reduce mortality in patients who had suffered from myocardial infarction (heart attack). In the study, 27 clinical centres randomized 1455 patients to receive encainide, flecainide, or placebo, while 272 were randomized to receive moricizine or placebo. In April 1989 the encainide, flecainide, placebo arm of the study was discontinued because of excess mortality in the experimental groups; 33 of 730 patients (4.5%) taking either encainide or flecainide had died after an average of 10 months follow-up, while only 9 of 725 patients (1.2%) taking placebo had died from arrhythmia and non-fatal cardiac arrest over

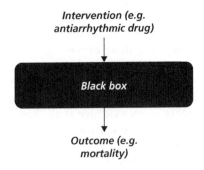

Figure 10.1 Comparative clinical research.

the same time period [112]. The experimental drugs also accounted for higher total mortality (56 of 730, or 7.7% versus 22 of 725 or 3.0%). Similar negative results were soon found for moricizine [113].

The essential feature of comparative clinical studies for present purposes is that the mechanism describing *how* the intervention caused the outcome is, as far as the study is concerned, a "black box" (Figure 10.1). As we saw in earlier chapters, the main problem with comparative clinical studies is that we are never certain whether we have ruled out all confounding factors. The current view is that using large numbers of study participants, randomization, concealed allocation, blinding (masking) [405], intention to treat, and (sometimes) the use of placebo controls reduce the likelihood of confounding. While these strategies can be legitimately criticized, the techniques for reducing confounding are, on the whole, correct. In fact, a theme of this chapter is that while much effort has been spent over the last several decades researching the methodology of comparative clinical studies, the methodology and quality of mechanistic reasoning has been altogether ignored.

In contrast with comparative clinical studies, mechanistic reasoning involves looking "inside the black box" at what happens to the relevant mechanisms affected by an intervention. A problem with understanding mechanistic reasoning is that the term "mechanism" has several meanings. Consider the following definitions from the recent literature:

Mechanisms are entities and activities organized such that they are productive of regular changes from start or set-up to finish or termination conditions [401].

A mechanism underlying a behaviour is a complex system which produces that behaviour by the interaction of a number of parts according to direct causal laws [399].

A mechanism is a structure performing a function in virtue of its component parts, component operations, and their organization. The orchestrated functioning of the mechanism is responsible for one or more phenomena [390].

A nomological machine[9] is a stable enough arrangement of components whose features acting in consort give rise to (relatively) stable input/output relations. Most, if not all, causal laws, hold only locally, relative to a nomological machine that ensures them. For example, a car lever, when pressed, makes a car accelerate. This is a stable law, but only acts locally (in cars, trucks etc.) – it does not apply to just any old lever. The nomological machine (the engine and other relevant components) guarantees that in the case of the *car* the lever controls acceleration [54].

There are interesting potential problems [406], and important differences between these definitions. At the same time, there is significant common ground (I am grateful to Nancy Cartwright for pointing out these similarities). With this in mind, With that in mind, I will adopt the following characterization of mechanisms that all mechanistic philosophers might all agree captures the essence of what they all mean individually by "mechanisms":

Mechanisms: are arrangements of parts/features that (allegedly) ensure a regular relationship between "inputs" and "outputs."

The heart (as a pump), the brain (as a control centre), and the liver (as a detoxifying agent, among other things) are all mechanisms in this sense.

However descriptions of mechanisms, by themselves, even if true descriptions, do not count as evidence. To count as evidence for claims that interventions have their putative patient-relevant effects, we must infer *from* (supposed) knowledge of the relevant mechanisms *to* claims that treatments have patient-relevant effects. In order for this inference to be acceptable, we must know what happens to each of the relevant mechanisms under intervention. Consider a rather famous case of mechanistic evidence involving antiarrhythmic drugs to reduce mortality in patients who had suffered myocardial infarction (heart attack). Myocardial infarction often damages the muscle and electrical system in the heart, leaving it susceptible to arrhythmias. A common type of arrhythmia, ventricular extra beats (VEBs), occurs when the left ventricle contracts before it has had time to fill completely. The heart then fails to pump sufficient blood. Without treatment, lung, brain, and kidney damage ensues. Worse, VEBs can also degenerate into ventricular fibrillation, or complete electrical chaos. Sudden death soon follows ventricular fibrillation in the absence of electric shock[8]. Large-scale epidemiological studies suggested that between 25 and 50% of sudden cardiac deaths were associated with arrhythmias [407–409]. Based on this understanding of the underlying mechanisms, several drugs were developed and found to be successful for regulating

---

[8]I am grateful to Jeffrey Aronson for careful explanation of the details of the mechanism of antiarrhythmic drugs.

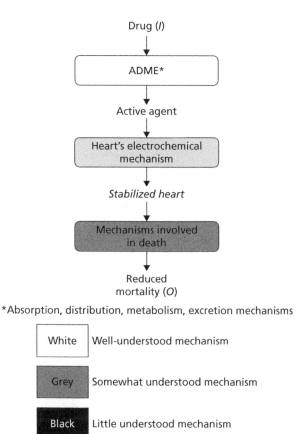

Figure 10.2 Mechanisms involved in antiarrhythmic drug action.

VEBs [410,411]. The drugs became widely prescribed in the belief that they would reduce cardiac deaths.

The mechanism(s) involved in antiarrhythmic drug action (Figure 10.2) might include swallowing and gastric emptying, metabolizing, circulatory, and binding mechanisms. The mechanisms involved in getting the orally administered drug to its pharmacological targets on the cells are relatively (but not completely) well understood and referred to in the medical literature as ADME (mechanisms for absorption, distribution, metabolism, and excretion). Once the drug reaches its cellular target, antiarrhythmic drugs reduce the frequency of VEBs by modifying the heart's electro-chemical mechanism. Finally, a reduction in VEBs (allegedly) reduces the risk of sudden death. If we accept the current definition of death as sustained lack of electrical activity in the brain, the reduction in mortality can be explained by brain mechanism(s).

Mechanistic reasoning involves *inferring* from the knowledge of the mechanism(s) to the claim that an intervention has its putative effects. I might know about the ADME, heart, and brain mechanisms, but to move from there to the claim that an antiarrhythmic drug will reduce mortality, I must be able to predict what happens to each of the mechanisms under intervention[9]. With this in mind, mechanistic reasoning can be defined as follows:

Mechanistic reasoning: involves an inference from mechanisms to claims that an intervention produces a patient-relevant outcome. Such reasoning will involve an inferential chain linking the intervention (such as antiarrhythmic drugs) with a clinical outcome (such as mortality).

Sound mechanistic reasoning requires that we establish what happens to each relevant mechanism under intervention. Such knowledge will inevitably involve an inferential chain or web linking the medical intervention with the patient-relevant outcomes (Figure 10.2).

An important feature of mechanistic reasoning in clinical medicine is that it must include mechanism(s) pertinent to patient-relevant outcomes. In brief, a patient-relevant outcome is one that makes people feel better or live longer. I will argue below that one reason for the over-confidence in mechanistic reasoning is that relatively simple biological [401] or physical [54] mechanisms have generally been considered. While these relatively simple mechanisms are undoubtedly important links in the pathway(s) linking a medical intervention and, say, death, they are rarely sufficient to conclude anything substantial about the relationship between an intervention and a patient-relevant outcome.

Another important feature of mechanistic reasoning as I have construed it is that it does not rely on the choice mechanisms one chooses

---

[9]We must also assume causal transitivity [412–414]. The following type of case might suggest that causes in clinical medicine are not necessarily transitive. A patient hears dull voices, and a psychiatrist mistakenly diagnoses her patient with manic depression (in fact, the "patient" had merely heard strange but real voices from a neighbour's house). The diagnosis makes the patient anxious and, in turn, causes the patient's symptoms to worsen. The patient is hospitalized, medicated, and counselled. After a year the patient no longer hears dull voices. However, it turns out that the patient would have recovered within a year had he not seen anyone (or had the psychiatrist not prescribed hospitalization, medication, and counselling). Here too, the diagnosis led to hospitalization, which in turn caused recovery, but it seems strange to assert that the diagnosis caused the recovery since the patient would have recovered in the same time without the hospitalization and diagnosis.

to describe. For example, since most mechanisms in the body involve the central nervous system, we might have linked the central nervous system to the various mechanisms in the example. Then, it is almost always possible to redescribe the mechanism in terms of lower-level mechanisms. In the example above, we might have included some of the heart's cellular mechanisms in our description. The essential feature of mechanistic reasoning is that it involves an inferential chain or web linking the intervention with the patient-relevant outcome via the relevant mechanisms. The "quality" of the mechanistic reasoning will then depend on the extent to which we can establish what happens to these relevant mechanisms under intervention.

One might object that I have conflated epistemological with ontological issues. Complete knowledge of all relevant mechanisms, people could insist, *is* sufficient to count as evidence. The problem, they say, is that we do not have sufficient knowledge of the mechanisms. Claude Bernard, perhaps the grandfather of contemporary mechanistic reasoning, expressed this view quite clearly. Understanding mechanisms, to Bernard, supposedly provided us with stable, even deterministic laws that did away with the need for any further "empirical" evidence:

> Now that the cause of the itch is known and experimentally determined, it has all become scientific, and empiricism has disappeared. We know the tick, and by it we explain the transmission of the itch, the skin changes and the cure, which is only the tick's death through appropriate application of toxic agents. . . .We cure it *always* without any exception, when we place ourselves in the known experimental conditions for reaching this goal [9].

Expressing what might be interpreted as a contemporary version of a similar view, Cartwright states:

> When a. . .nomological machine [mechanism] obtains, there will not only be a stable causal law, but there will also be a *reason* why the law is stable and in many cases we can recognize when this reason holds and when not and what kinds of manipulations will jeopardize it [53].

I have two responses to this objection. First, my aim is to deal with an epistemological rather than an ontological problem. I do not wish to deny that there are underlying mechanisms that could, in principle, provide complete explanations for how medical interventions work. However, if our knowledge of mechanisms is to count as reliable *evidence*, we need to know enough about the relevant mechanisms to predict how they will react to novel medical interventions. Second, the epistemological and ontological issues are intertwined. Even if we knew everything about the underlying mechanisms, in order for such knowledge to be useful, the mechanisms must have the fundamental property of behaving predictably under intervention if they are to provide the basis for reliable evidence. We will see in the next section that our knowledge of mechanisms is often lacking, and that our predictions to what happens to mechanisms under intervention is mistaken, sometimes leading to tragic medical errors. There are two explanations for these commonly mistaken predictions. First, it could be epistemological and we simply do not know enough about the relevant mechanisms, in which case mechanistic reasoning is unlikely to provide reliable evidence. Second, the problem could be metaphysical and mechanisms themselves do not underwrite stable and predictable input–output relationships. In both cases mechanistic reasoning is problematic.

With the definitions out of the way I will now argue that, contrary to what Russo and Williamson assert, mechanistic reasoning is *not* required to establish causal claims.

10.3 Why the strong view that mechanistic reasoning is necessary to establish causal claims is mistaken

Russo and Williamson's claim that "two different types of evidence – probabilistic and mechanistic – are at stake when deciding whether or not to accept a causal claim" [403]. They support their claim with two arguments, one "historical" and the other "theoretical." I will contend that neither stands up to scrutiny.

10.3.1 Russo and Williamson's "historical" argument that mechanistic reasoning is required to support causal claims

Russo and Williamson note that antisepsis, *Helicobacter pylori*, and the link between smoking and lung cancer, although supported by strong evidence from comparative clinical research, were not accepted until their mechanisms were understood:

> The history of medicine presents many cases in which causal claims made solely on the basis of statistics have been rejected until backed by mechanistic or theoretical knowledge. For instance, in 19th-century Austria, the risk of puerperal fever after childbirth was extremely serious. . . . In spite of the extensive statistics gathered corroborating this

hypothesis, Semmelweis' claim about cadaverical contamination and puerperal fever was accepted only after the germ theory of disease was developed [403].

However, in the historical examples Russo and Williamson cite, the demand for mechanistic evidence (in addition to high-quality comparative clinical studies) before causation was supposedly established delayed the adoption of life-saving interventions. One might appeal to the very same examples to argue that it is unwise to require mechanistic reasoning alongside strong evidence from comparative clinical studies. Indeed Gillies [89], whom Russo and Williamson cite as a source for these examples, argues just this:

> . . .it becomes obvious that any new practice which can be shown statistically to be better than alternative practices as regards either prevention or cure, and which does not have any harmful side-effects, should be adopted [89].

Russo (in correspondence) admits that in the absence of a confirmed mechanism, one should act in light of strong comparative clinical studies. However, if, as Russo and Williamson appear to argue, mechanistic reasoning is required to establish causal claims, then it is reasonable to *doubt* the causal claim supported by the strong comparative clinical studies. Indeed this is just what skeptics about Semmelweis' proposal argued. My argument is that mechanistic reasoning is *not* necessary to establish causal claims.

Another defense that Russo and Williamson might use is that their thesis is a description of what happened in order for certain hypotheses to be adopted:

> It is worth pointing out that we are not concerned, here, with how scientists came up with (controversial) causal hypotheses. . . but rather with *how those hypotheses have become accepted by the medical community*. . .what matters is that this *claim was not accepted* until backed up by mechanistic evidence, i.e., until the germ theory had been developed [403].

Yet their account fails as a general description. While it is true that in the Semmelweis case (and a few others) mechanistic reasoning was required before the medical community accepted a hypothesis, there are many other examples where treatments were widely accepted before any semblance of

a mechanism was established. To name a few, Percival Pott's hypothesis
that soot caused scrotum cancer (1775) was accepted years before benzpy-
rene was identified (1933), Edward Jenner introduced smallpox vaccines
(1798) decades before anyone really understood how they worked, John
Snow helped eliminate cholera with cleaner water (1849) years before the
Vibrio cholerae was identified (1893), and Carlos Finlay reduced the rates
of yellow fever by killing mosquitoes (1881) decades before flavivirus was
identified (1927). In the last century, general anesthesia, aspirin, and steroids were widely used for decades before their mechanisms were understood. In this century, deep brain stimulation has been used to suppress
tremors in patients with advanced Parkinson's disease, and also to cure
other motor function disorders such as dystonia or Tourette's syndrome,
yet researchers have not been able to identify its mechanism of action with
any certainty[10]. In fact, the case against the view that the medical community requires mechanistic reasoning before accepting a hypothesis can be
made much more strongly. The antiarrhythmic example, and at least 17
others (see Appendix), indicate that, historically, the medical community
often views high-quality comparative clinical studies as sufficient even in
the face of *conflicting* mechanistic reasoning.

More importantly, Russo and Williamson state in other places that they
are attempting to do more than describe: "Our point...is a theoretical but
not an historical one" [403]. Before discussing this "theoretical" argument
in more detail, I will consider a weaker version of the claim that mechanistic evidence is required alongside statistical evidence before accepting a
hypothesis. The weaker claim is that special subsets of hypotheses, namely
apparently implausible ones, require mechanistic evidence before they
should be accepted even if they are strongly supported by comparative
clinical studies.

Consider the following example of an implausible hypothesis supported
by a comparative clinical study. In July 2000, 3393 patients who had been
admitted to hospital between 1990 and 1996 were randomized to control
and treatment groups. A remote, retroactive, intercessory prayer was said
for the well-being and full recovery of the intervention group [415]. The
results indicated that although mortality (deaths) were the same in intervention and control groups, "[l]ength of stay in hospital and duration of
fever were significantly shorter in the intervention group than in the control group ($P = 0.01$ and $P = 0.04$, respectively)" [415].

If we take randomized trials to provide "gold standard" evidence, it
seems that we should advocate retroactive prayer as an effective, simple,

[10]I am grateful to Rafaela Campaner and Maria Carla Galavotti for bringing many of
these examples to my attention.

and cheap intervention without any known adverse effects for reducing stay in the hospital and duration of fever. At the same time, the Leibovici study seems implausible because it confronts the widely held principle that causes precede their effects. Any hypothesis that relies on a mechanism whereby causes precede their effects can therefore (on this view) be rejected out of hand.

One way to interpret the rejection of the Leibovici study on mechanistic grounds is as an appeal to the principle of total evidence, namely that no relevant evidence should be ignored. On this view, mechanistic reasoning should be weighed alongside any other evidence when deciding whether to accept or reject a hypothesis. Since the "mechanistic reasoning" indicates that remote retroactive prayer does not have effects, it should be weighed (and, in this case, *outweigh*) other competing evidence. Indeed a central thesis of this chapter is that *high-quality* mechanistic reasoning should be weighed alongside results from comparative clinical studies.

Yet there are reasons to be cautious about using mechanistic reasoning to rule out or reduce our confidence in apparently implausible results from comparative clinical studies; moreover, the principle of total evidence does not imply that we *require* mechanistic reasoning to rule out implausible hypotheses.

For one, such a strategy might also have rejected Semmelweis and Marshall's hypotheses. One could defend the strategy by arguing that Leibovici's hypothesis is far less plausible than Semmelweis' or Marshall's. While such a defence is possible – indeed I will suggest one along these lines in section 10.3.2 – it is not as easy at is appears to distinguish between shades of plausibility. It seems that many people are more likely to believe claims about therapeutic effects that are explained by (apparently) plausible mechanisms and more likely to be skeptical about such claims when they are not supported by plausible mechanisms. However, the Semmelweis example suggests that our psychological skepticism in the face of high-quality evidence from comparative clinical studies should be tempered, while the example of sudden infant death syndrome (SIDS) and others from the Appendix suggest that we should be more skeptical about therapeutic claims that are supported by apparently plausible mechanisms *without* high-quality evidence from comparative clinical studies.

More importantly, the principle of total evidence does not imply that we require mechanistic reasoning to rule out implausible hypotheses that are supported by comparative clinical studies. Sometimes close examination of the comparative clinical study itself is sufficient. While Semmelweis' comparative clinical study produced a dramatic result, the Leibovici study was questionable on several grounds. The main outcome, mortality, was *higher* (although not statistically significantly) in the group that was prayed for. Then, it is unclear whether the outcomes that appeared to be positively affected by retroactive prayer were specified in advance. Eyebrows should immediately be raised when investigators report the effects of the experimental intervention on several secondary outcomes without specifying them in advance. The nature of classical hypothesis testing means that if we measure enough outcomes, we are likely to find some that differ *statistically* (but not necessarily relevantly) between groups due to chance alone. Failure to specify whether the outcomes were chosen in advance leaves the possibility that Leibovici considered dozens of potential outcomes until he found some that were significantly different in both groups due to chance alone.

Finally, the effect size in the Leibovici study was minuscule. Leibovici reports the median and interquartile range (in days) of the length of stay in hospital and duration of fever. The median for the duration of fever was the same in both groups (2 days). What accounted for the apparent effects of retroactive prayer to reduce fever was the tiny difference in interquartile ranges (1–4 for the intervention group and 1–5 for the control group). The median for the length of stay in hospital was 8 days (interquartile range 4–13) for the intervention group and 7 days (interquartile range 4–16) for the control group. As argued earlier, small absolute differences must be interpreted with caution because they can be confounded by small, often undetected bias. In short, Leibovici's trial does not support the hypothesis that remote retroactive prayer has any effects.

I have not chosen these methodological flaws with the Leibovici study *ad hoc*. The problem with multiple endpoints is well recognized [416,417]. Meanwhile, there are independent, although perhaps insufficiently recognized, reasons for being far more wary about the increased danger of confounding with small effects [140,178,418].

In short we do not *require* mechanistic reasoning to remain skeptical about conclusions from comparative clinical studies. In cases where the comparative clinical studies are not of high quality, we can remain skeptical about any hypothesis it supports.

10.3.2 Russo and Williamson's "theoretical" argument

In addition to the "historical" argument, Russo and Williamson also have what they dub a "theoretical" argument: "if there is no plausible mechanism from C to E, then any correlation is likely to be spurious" [403]. Making a similar claim, Glennan states:

> It is a truism that correlation is not causation, but attempts to spell
> out what distinguishes causal correlations from accidental ones

have not been particularly successful. MTC [mechanical theory of causation] meets this deficiency by requiring that two events are causally related if and only if those events are connected by a mechanism [419].

These quotes suggest that Russo and Williamson (and others) advocate the view that mechanistic reasoning is *required* alongside comparative clinical studies to rule out spurious correlations. This is certainly how Gillies [404] interprets them. They may, of course, be making a weaker claim, namely that mechanistic evidence reduces the chances that a correlation is spurious. However, because Russo and Williamson may be making the stronger claim, and it may seem plausible given the ontological importance many take mechanisms to have, I will rehearse arguments against it.

It is true that comparative clinical studies sometimes support spurious relationships, and that all hypotheses are underdetermined by evidence. To borrow Russo and Williamson's own example, we might find that there are more storks in areas where the birth rate is highest, and mistakenly conclude that the storks caused the increase in birth rate.

However the Semmelweis and *Helicobacter pylori* cases are counterexamples to the claim that mechanistic reasoning generally rules out spurious relationships. The Appendix contains 17 other examples where high-quality comparative clinical studies were used to overturn spurious hypotheses that had been supported by mechanistic reasoning. However, it is not my aim here to argue for the superiority of high-quality comparative clinical studies over high-quality mechanistic reasoning (or vice versa), which would require a detailed independent investigation. That being said, a theme of this chapter is that while the methodology of comparative clinical studies has been investigated for decades, standards for mechanistic reasoning have yet to be provided. Hence, we have (albeit imperfect) criteria for evaluating the quality of comparative clinical studies, while, as the above examples suggest, the reliability of mechanistic reasoning has been left to hand-waving.

Moreover, some comparative clinical studies, notably randomized trials, are quite good at ruling out spurious relationships. For example, if we were to ignore ethical and practical constraints, and randomize couples to live close or far from storks, we would probably find that there was no difference in birth rates.

One might alter the claim that mechanistic reasoning is required to rule out spurious relationships and argue instead that hypotheses supported by both comparative clinical studies and mechanistic reasoning are less likely to be spurious than hypotheses supported by one type of evidence alone. Such a claim might rest on the plausible premise that since each type of evidence suffers from different potential pitfalls, a hypothesis supported by both types of evidence is less likely to have been confounded. This weaker claim is altogether acceptable and indeed underwritten by the principle of total evidence. However, in its altered form it can no longer be interpreted as Russo and Williamson's thesis.

To sum up, neither the "historical" or "theoretical" arguments of Russo and Williamson support the view that mechanistic reasoning is required alongside comparative clinical studies. The historical examples, even those cited by Russo and Williamson, indicate that many lives would have been saved had the requirement for mechanistic reasoning been dropped in cases where we had evidence from high-quality comparative clinical studies. Then, the notion that mechanistic reasoning rules out spurious relationships is mistaken.

10.4 Two epistemological problems with mechanistic reasoning

There are two common and related problems with mechanistic reasoning. Both are epistemological. First, biochemical mechanisms upon which the mechanisms are based are rarely sufficiently well understood to predict how they will behave under intervention. Second, the inferential chain (or, perhaps more accurately, web) linking the intervention with the patient-relevant outcome via the relevant mechanisms is generally more complex than is appreciated. These problems often make mechanistic reasoning unreliable as a source of evidence that medical interventions have their putative patient-relevant effects. In this section I will describe the problems in detail and explain why the problems are, and are likely to remain, common.

10.4.1 The first problem with mechanistic reasoning: unknown mechanisms

Some medical historians have suggested that until at least 1860, and probably 1940, most medical interventions were no better than placebo or positively harmful [290,349]. These useless or harmful treatments were often justified on (bogus) mechanistic grounds. For example, Galen (AD 129–200) thought that blood was created and used up rather than circulated, so bloodletting was a way of releasing blood that was stagnating in the extremities. It follows that releasing the stagnating blood somehow caused alleviation of various symptoms. Bloodletting was also justified by the theory of the four humors[11]. Blood was seen to be the dominant humor and most in need of control. According to this theory, letting blood caused the humors to become balanced once again. Although bloodletting may have made patients feel better in the short term, there is little doubt that it caused a worsening of many of the ailments it was used to treat. We now know that the humoral theory is mistaken – blood circulates rather than being used up. I refer to mechanisms that do not have any valuable empirical support as "empty." Mechanistic reasoning based on empty mechanism is (obviously) unlikely to be reliable. It seems fair to say that had these therapies been submitted to comparative clinical studies they would have been exposed as useless or harmful.

Although our current understanding of physiological and pathological mechanisms has come a long way since the days when bloodletting was common, the temptation to accept treatments justified by (practically) empty mechanisms remains. Dr Benjamin Spock, for example, had a seductive rationale for placing babies to sleep on their stomachs to reduce infant mortality:

> There are two disadvantages to a baby's sleeping on his back. If he vomits he's more likely to choke on the vomitus. Also he tends to keep his head turned toward the same side. . .this may flatten the side of the head. . .I think it is preferable to accustom a baby to sleeping on his stomach from the start [421].

Dr Spock's advice, based on what seemed to be sound mechanisms for infant mortality, was widely followed. His bestselling book, *Baby and Child Care*, was published in numerous editions between 1946 and 1998, and sold over 50 million copies[12].

Beginning in the 1980s, however, comparative studies found a strong correlation between sleeping position and SIDS. Contrary to what Dr Spock's mechanistic reasoning suggested, significantly more babies who slept on their backs survived [422–427]. The plausibility of the studies was

---

[11]Humorism was an ancient Greek theory stating that the body was made up of four substances, black bile, yellow bile, phlegm, and blood. Diseases were thought to result from an imbalance of these humors. Interestingly, bloodletting continued long after the humoral theory of the body fell into disuse. Sir William Osler even recommended bloodletting in the 1919 and 1923 editions of his textbook *The Principles and Practice of Medicine* [420].

[12]Spock advocated back sleeping up to the 1955 (2nd) edition, but front sleeping from the 1956 edition onwards.

further supported by the fact that rates of SIDS dropped from roughly 0.6 per 1000 to 0.3 per 1000 in the USA and the UK, where campaigns to get babies sleeping on their backs have been successful[13]. Moreover, SIDS rates have historically been very low in countries where babies traditionally sleep on their backs [429,430]. In addition, the relationship between sleeping position and SIDS becomes stronger when adjustments are made for confounding factors [431–433].

In fact, there is currently no evidence that babies sleeping on their backs are more likely to choke on their own vomit. Healthy babies, unlike drunk or drugged adults, are quite skilled at swallowing and spitting. In short, Dr Spock had not identified the relevant mechanisms for SIDS and hence his reasoning was mistaken.

Related problems arise when some (but not all) of the relevant mechanisms involved in mechanistic reasoning are not based on sound evidence. This was the problem with the reasoning in the antiarrhythmic drug example. While researchers were relatively certain about what happened to the drugs when they were swallowed and even their effect on the heart's electrical mechanism, the impact of the drugs on mortality (the brain's electrochemical mechanism) was not based on sound evidence. The available evidence suggested an epidemiological association between VEBs and mortality, but association is not causation [434]. Moreover, even at the time there were good reasons to believe that after myocardial infarction, the heart is damaged in a way that both causes VEBs and raises the risk of sudden death. If this latter hypothesis had been taken more seriously, researchers might have predicted that intervening on a damaged heart could increase mortality.

A problem with mechanistic reasoning involving some empty mechanisms well known to the medical profession arises when researchers choose convenient surrogates (such as reduction in VEBs) for the desired outcome (such as mortality). When we use a surrogate outcome we assume, at the very least, that we understand what will happen to the further mechanism(s) responsible for the patient-relevant outcome under intervention. In the antiarrhythmic example, we assume what will happen to the brain's electrical mechanism after the heart's rhythm has been regulated. Unfortunately, what happens to the further mechanisms had not been established by reliable evidence [435–443].

---

[13]It has been estimated that at least 50 000 excess deaths occurred due to the bad advice in the USA alone in the period 1974–1991 [428]. To put these numbers into context, less than 60 000 Americans died in the Vietnam War, and less than 6000 Americans have died in the War on Terror since September 11, 2001 (including those who died in the 9/11 attacks).

When it comes to drug therapy, mechanistic reasoning is bound to be based on "partial" mechanisms because of the complexity and somewhat mysterious metabolic mechanism (Figure 10.3). The diagram in Figure 10.3 is accompanied by 49 explanatory notes including the following: "It is still unknown, if methyl oxidation at ring B occurs before or after esterification with phytol," "In some microorganisms, cystathionine synthesis takes place via O-acetyl-L-homoserine" and "This reaction may also occur with the 26-hydoxylated compound" [444]. The uncertainty of the metabolic mechanism means of course we cannot be sure what happens to what we swallow. This makes any accurate prediction about what happens to the metabolic mechanism (and therefore what happens to other relevant mechanisms) when an agent is introduced to the stomach difficult.

Like a chain with some weak links, or an argument with some weak premises, mechanistic reasoning based on partially understood mechanisms will not provide reliable evidence that an intervention caused a patient-relevant outcome. Indeed partial mechanisms often lead to more serious harm than empty mechanisms because their (albeit incomplete) empirical basis lends an aura of acceptability, which in turn leads to more prolific use

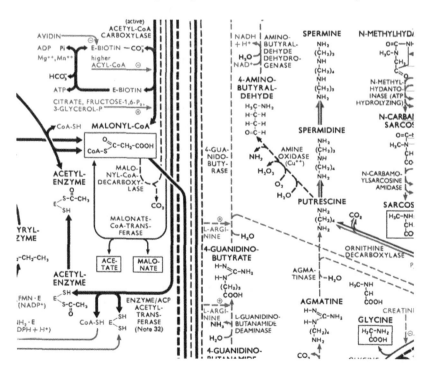

Figure 10.3 Small extract of metabolic mechanisms.

of a harmful treatment. This was certainly the case in the antiarrhythmic drug example. At the peak of their use over 200000 people were taking the drugs in the USA alone. Assuming that the results of the comparative clinical study were accurate, the drugs killed an estimated 10000 people in the USA alone. Worldwide, it has been estimated that they killed more people every year than were killed in action during the whole of the Vietnam War [24].

10.4.2 The second problem with mechanistic reasoning: stochastic and complex mechanisms

The next problem with mechanistic reasoning is that most interventions activate many, often unexpected, mechanisms, often probabilistically, making inferences from mechanisms to claims about efficacy precarious.

Biochemical mechanisms are almost always stochastic[14] [398,400] and complex. For example, the mechanism for how smoking increases the risk of lung cancer is relatively well understood yet not all smokers contract lung cancer, nor are all lung cancers caused by smoking. Even quantum mechanics, perhaps our most empirically successful theory, is intrinsically stochastic, in that it assigns probabilities to the values of measurement outcomes. For example, it assigns a probability of 0.5 to the outcome of a measurement of the "spin" of an electron (in a particular "direction").

For example, the link between flecainide and reduction in VEBs (via the swallowing, metabolic, and heart mechanisms) was gathered from small comparative clinical studies that suggested a success rate of about 90% [410,411]. Then (setting aside the fact that this was merely an association) the evidence for the link between VEBs and sudden cardiac death (via the heart and brain mechanisms) was gathered from large-scale epidemiological studies that suggested that 25–50% of sudden cardiac deaths are due to arrhythmias [407–409]. If we assume independence, the strength of the overall relationship between antiarrhythmic drug therapy and mortality will be the product of the strengths of the individual relationships. However, it is unreasonable to assume independence, which adds to the problem of estimating the effect size suggested by mechanistic reasoning.

Provided, of course, that we had sufficient knowledge of what happened to the mechanisms in a pathway linking the drug therapy with mortality,

---

[14]Determinist supporters of mechanistic reasoning such as Claude Bernard would, of course, insist that probabilistic behavior is merely indicative that further research must be done to bring apparently probabilistic processes into line. But whether or not we shall someday discover underlying deterministic laws is beside the point. At present (and the foreseeable future) even mechanisms involving fundamental particles, and *a fortiori* for higher-level entities such as cells, organs, and biological relations, are probabilistic rather than deterministic.

it might seem reasonable to infer *some* dependency of the outcome on the intervention (even if the failure to assume independence made it difficult to estimate its precise strength). But recall from Chapter 3 that in order to determine whether a treatment's benefits outweigh its harms, we require an estimate of its absolute effect size. Most interventions activate a complex web of biochemical mechanisms that make such an inference precarious.

As an illustration, consider one type of complexity known as a *paradoxical* response, whereby the same drug has one effect in some cases and the opposite effect in others, presumably by activating different mechanisms, or at least by causing a different response in the same mechanism (Figure 10.4). Philosophers have discussed these examples for decades; perhaps the best known, due to Hesslow (1976) is the case of birth control pills causing increased risk of thrombosis but decreasing the risk of pregnancy (which itself increases the risk of thrombosis). Hence the same intervention (birth control pills) can both increase and decrease the risk of thrombosis [251,445,446].

Recently, Hauben and Aronson [447] have listed no fewer than 67 drugs that sometimes worsen the condition for which they are indicated. To name a few, opioids can both reduce and increase pain [448,449] and antidepressants can both reduce and worsen depressive symptoms [450,451]. Even the same molecule can initiate very different mechanisms depending on its environment within the body. Indeed the "one-many" phenomenon is considered to be a robust empirical generalization [452–454]. Or, in the case of antiarrhythmic drugs, it was well known at the outset that the drugs *increased* arrhythmias in about 11% of patients [455].

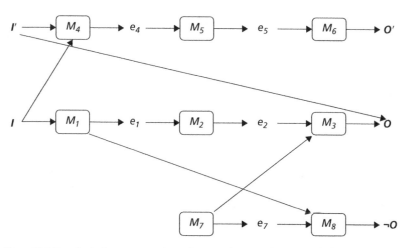

Figure 10.4 Paradoxical responses where the same intervention, *I*, can help (*O*) and harm (¬*O*) the same disorder, and outcomes that are caused by more than one cause (*I* and *I'*).

Less dramatic than paradoxical responses, interventions often produce unexpected harmful side-effects, again presumably by activating an additional mechanism(s) in some unexpected way. Perhaps the most infamous case of a drug with an unexpected side-effect was thalidomide, which was prescribed to cure the symptoms of morning sickness but which was later found to cause severe birth defects. It would be a misuse of language to say that thalidomide was effective. Unexpected side-effects can also be positive. For example, sildenafil was originally designed to cure hypertension (high blood pressure). However, the first clinical trials of the drug found it to be ineffective for hypertension, but quite effective at producing erections. The drug was marketed as Viagra and quickly became a huge commercial success.

Unexpected effects of placebos also illustrate how interventions can activate unsuspected mechanisms in relevant ways. In one example, olive and corn oil were used in placebo controls for cholesterol-lowering drugs before it was known that these oils had cholesterol-lowering properties of their own. Beatrice Golomb cites other similar examples:

> Sugar pills may affect blood insulin levels with their cascade of physiological effects, and a lactose "placebo" reportedly led to increased dropout rates in the control group in a study of patients with [HIV]; similarly, lactose placebos were a possible source of markedly increased gastrointestinal side effects in the placebo group in a study of patients with cancer. Subjects may react to excipients, stabilizers, dyes, or other elements, and I have cared for one patient whose painful unilateral neuropathy symptoms were ultimately traced – in repeated n-of-1 blinded comparison – to magnesium stearate, a common lubricant in pill formulation [272].

If supposedly "inactive" substances sometimes have positive or negative unanticipated effects on unexpected mechanisms that ultimately affect the target disorder, then *a fortiori* "active" substances will also sometimes surprise us.

Paradoxical responses and unexpected side-effects of both placebos and active substances are not the only type of complexity. The same phenomenon can be produced by many different causes, perhaps via different mechanisms, or at least mechanisms that can operate very differently. Hypertension (high blood pressure), depression, cancer, and many other ailments have more than one cause. Indeed, Broadbent [456] recently argued that the very idea of single causes of diseases is unlikely to apply outside infectious disease and diseases of deficiency.

To recap what has been discussed in this section, the probabilistic and complex nature of mechanisms suggests that our knowledge of underlying causal mechanisms will rarely provide a sound basis for predictions about the patient-relevant benefits of interventions. The stochastic relationship between the "inputs" and "outputs" of most medical mechanisms makes it difficult to estimate the size of an overall effect, and the often unanticipated complexity of the pathways linking the intervention and patient-relevant outcome make it problematic to estimate the direction of the overall effect (positive or negative).

Stuart Glennan (in correspondence) objected that the problems I have outlined with mechanistic reasoning are not problems with the mechanisms *per se* but rather epistemological problems with our knowledge of the mechanisms.

In response, Glennan is correct to insist that the problems I have identified with mechanistic reasoning do not imply that higher-level correlations are not realized in some way by the lower-level cellular and molecular entities and their interactions. At the same time, the limits to our understanding of the web of mechanisms that link a medical intervention and patient-relevant outcomes present serious problems for mechanistic reasoning.

Moreover, even if we had perfect knowledge of underlying mechanisms, in order to be useful for predictions about how interventions affect patient-relevant outcomes, Glennan would have to assume that the mechanisms themselves produce *stable* input–output relationships. While it is safe to assume that many mechanisms do behave predictably, it is far from clear whether the assumption of stability holds in general. Many philosophers of science (including those mentioned above) *define* mechanisms as productive of stable input–output relationships, such stability must be established rather than defined into existence.

In spite of the serious and often under-recognized problems with mechanistic reasoning, EBM proponents are perhaps too quick to dismiss all mechanistic reasoning as equally problematic. I will now argue that some mechanistic reasoning is sufficiently free from the problems listed above to count as strong evidence for the putative effects of medical interventions.

10.5 Why EBM proponents should allow a more prominent role for high-quality (valid and based on "complete" mechanisms) mechanistic reasoning in their evidence hierarchies

Just as we will never be completely certain that all confounding factors have been ruled out in a comparative clinical study, we will never be certain that we have *complete* understanding of all potential mechanisms linking the intervention with patient-relevant outcomes. Hence, in the spirit of Fisher's hypothesis tests [198] and Popper's falsification [171], mechanistic reasoning should be judged on the extent to which it overcomes obvious flaws. Accordingly, mechanistic reasoning must satisfy the following desiderata that must be satisfied to count as of sufficiently high quality to provide strong evidence.

1 The knowledge of mechanisms upon which the mechanistic reasoning is based is *not incomplete*, i.e. there are no obvious gaps in our knowledge of the inferential chain linking the intervention and the patient-relevant outcome.

A not-incomplete understanding of the mechanistic chain linking the intervention with the clinically relevant outcome avoids obvious gaps such as those illustrated in the bloodletting, antiarrhythmic drug, and SIDS examples discussed above. Each link in the inferential chain should be based on sufficiently strong evidence, perhaps (but not necessarily) from high-quality comparative clinical studies. The second desideratum is that any mechanistic reasoning must factor in the complex and stochastic nature of most biochemical mechanisms.

2 The probabilistic and complex nature of the mechanisms are explicitly taken into account when inferring from mechanisms to any claims that a particular intervention has a patient-relevant benefit.

By "complex nature" I mean the other mechanisms that might get triggered by the intervention, and produce either undesirable side-effects or even paradoxical effects.

When the two desiderata have been met, the mechanistic reasoning in question can be judged to be of high quality and should count as strong evidence that a medical therapy will produce its putative patient-relevant outcome(s). While instances of high-quality mechanistic reasoning are rare, the following are real examples that can be used to challenge the EBM refusal to allow any role for mechanistic reasoning.

Large nodular goiters present an obstruction in the airway that impairs respiratory function. At the same time, there is strong evidence that radiotherapy shrinks goiter and that it is generally safe [457,458]. Then our knowledge about the mechanics of breathing (the mechanism) tells us that reducing the size of the airway obstruction will improve respiratory function. There is also strong evidence (from comparative clinical studies) that radiotherapy does not induce any paradoxical responses or severe harmful side-effects. In short, there are no obvious gaps in the mechanistic knowledge linking the intervention with the patient-relevant outcome, and the possibility of serious adverse events (complexity) was made unlikely by the clinical trials in the various stages of the inferential chain. Mechanistic reasoning should therefore allow us to conclude that radiotherapy will improve respiratory function, at least in the longer term (radiotherapy is known to induce short-term thyroid swelling). However, proponents of the view that mechanistic reasoning is *never* sufficient insisted on conducting a clinical trial of the effects of radiotherapy on goiter to improve respiratory function [459]. They found, perhaps unsurprisingly, that radiotherapy improved respiratory function. One might question whether the trial was justified (as far as it was used to test the hypothesis that respiratory function would improve) given the high-quality mechanistic reasoning. (This is yet another example where ethics and epistemology are intertwined [46,74].)

In another example, mechanistic reasoning provided solid evidence that an accelerated hepatitis B immunization schedule was as effective as the standard schedule. Conventional hepatitis B immunization schedules involve injections at 0, 1, and 6 months. The conventional regimen has proven effective at both long-term seroprotection (production and maintenance of antibodies) and immunity from hepatitis B virus (HBV) infection [460,461]. However, the conventional regimen is inconvenient for travellers who have to go to an HBV endemic area on short notice. An accelerated regimen, whereby injections are given at 0, 10, and 21 days, was studied in randomized trials and shown to result in the same high seroproduction rates as the regular regimen [462,463]. It has also been known for several decades that clinical hepatitis B is caused by HBV [464] and our general understanding of the immune system (a "mechanism") that the antibodies in the vaccine neutralize HBV [465–467]. It was concluded from the similar seroproduction rates that the accelerated regimen produced the same immunity as the longer regimen. The conclusion was not "not incomplete" in any plausible way, and it is reasonable to accept that the accelerated vaccination schedule produces immunity, at least in the short term.

These examples suggest that high-quality mechanistic reasoning can provide reliable evidence that a treatment is effective. It can be used (perhaps exceptionally) as sufficient support for hypotheses that medical interventions cause patient-relevant outcomes and, more generally, to strengthen the support of such hypotheses (Figure 10.5). EBM proponents, by failing to distinguish between high- and low-quality mechanistic reasoning, have overlooked an important and useful source of evidence.

Before considering whether mechanistic reasoning can be useful for generalizing the results of a study, it is important to note that the same criteria apply when we use mechanistic reasoning to *reject* a hypothesis. Low-quality mechanistic reasoning should not be admissible as evidence that a hypothesis is false, while high-quality mechanistic reasoning should be allowed to question the results from comparative clinical studies. It is beyond the scope of this work to conduct a detailed analysis, but it is reasonable to suspect that the mechanistic reasoning that led to the rejection of Semmelweis' hypothesis was of low quality, while the mechanistic reasoning used to question Leibovici's hypothesis was of high quality.

10.6 Mechanisms and other roles in clinical medicine

It's not that causes and their effects never instance natural regularities. It's just that causality is one thing, and regularity, another.

—J. Bogen [392]

In addition to being used as evidence for efficacy, some have argued that mechanisms are required for understanding [401], explanation [390,392], generalizing causal hypotheses [37,56], analyzing reasoning in discovery [390], unification [395], and for solving Hume's problem [399]. It is beyond the scope of this work to consider these other roles in any detail. However,

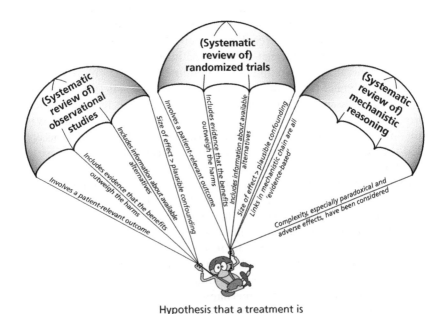

Figure 10.5 A picture is emerging: how mechanistic reasoning can be considered alongside evidence from randomized trials and observational studies.

two general comments apply. First, no matter what role mechanisms are purported to play, they must be of high quality as defined above; hence, the above analysis is relevant no matter what other roles mechanisms are to play. Second, even if mechanisms are useful in these other ways, my arguments about the limited role for mechanistic reasoning as evidence for efficacy or effectiveness stands. Moreover, I believe that the other roles for mechanisms have been overstated. I will limit myself here to a brief sketch of what I believe to be the problems with using mechanisms to generalize the results of clinical trials and to generate hypotheses.

10.6.1 Exposing the dogma that knowledge of mechanisms allows us to generalize the results of a study

Researchers have employed two distinct strategies employing mechanisms as a solution to the problem of external validity. The first, propounded by Russo and Williamson, Cartwright, Machamer, Darden, and Craver, and even the EBM movement itself, is that we understand *stable* mechanisms to justify the inference from average trial results to predictions of how individuals outside the trial will respond. The second, attributable to La Caze, contends that mechanism-derived subgroups solves the problem of external validity. I will argue that both are problematic: we rarely have enough information to confirm the stability of mechanisms across populations to be able to help generalize, and mechanisms are not required to define subgroups.

To Cartwright, once we have identified a mechanism, we are in a position to predict how an individual (or group) from outside the trial would react to the treatment. She illustrates her view with several examples, including the following one borrowed from Morrison:

> . . .let us say that an experiment is conducted to increase security and reduce theft in two schools through the introduction of closed circuit television (CCTV). The effect is a reduction in theft in the experimental school. Exactly what is the cause here? It may be that potential offenders are deterred from theft, or it might be that offenders are caught more frequently, or it might be that the presence of the CCTV renders teacher and students more vigilant [42].

If the mechanism by which CCTV lowers crime is that the cameras are visible, then the cameras should be placed in highly visible locations. Otherwise they won't work. Or, if the mechanism by which CCTV lowers crime is that police are quickly alerted, then we had better make sure that someone monitors the images from the cameras and notifies the police of any suspicious activity quickly.

Perhaps surprisingly, the EBM movement adopts a position very similar to Cartwright's:

> A sound understanding of pathophysiology [mechanisms] is necessary to interpret and apply the results of clinical research. For instance, most patients to whom we would like to generalize the results of randomized trials would, for one reason or another, not have been enrolled in the most relevant study. The patient may be too old, be too sick, have other underlying illnesses, or be uncooperative. Understanding the underlying pathophysiology allows the clinician to better judge whether the results are applicable to the patient at hand [12].

Gordon Guyatt and Paul Glasziou (in conversation) have offered the following illustration of the EBM view. A trial excludes everyone over the age of 60. Then, they ask whether the results of the trial will be applicable to a 61 year old, and also whether the results of the trial will be applicable to a 90 year old. They claim that mechanistic reasoning supports the view that the intervention is likely to work for the 61 year old, but unlikely to work for the 90 year old.

However, in order for mechanistic reasoning to help us generalize, we must make two strong and often unjustified assumptions. First, the reasoning must be of high quality (as defined above), and second we must assume that the mechanisms operating in the study population operate in the same way as the mechanisms operating in the individual who presents him or herself to the practice.

I will not examine either of these assumptions in detail here, but satisfy myself by pointing out how the assumptions are not justified as often as many have assumed. Neither the examples used by Cartwright nor the EBM movement are cases of high-quality mechanistic reasoning as they stand. The proposed mechanisms for how CCTV reduces crime (deterrence or vigilance) are empty in that they are based on mere conjecture: what is the evidence that the mechanisms are deterrence or vigilance? CCTV might also work because the thieving students saw them being installed and notified their colleagues to stop stealing until they thought of a new plan. It is also possible that installing CCTV could instigate a paradoxical response. The CCTV cameras might make students feel criminalized, and goad them into behaving more badly.

In a similar vein, the Glasziou/Guyatt example relies on a hidden simplifying assumption that the mechanism is (in some unspecified way) age sensitive. If the mechanism were age sensitive, then a treatment that

worked in a 60 year old is likely to work in a 61 year old. But the simplifying assumption is unwarranted. The mechanism might be sensitive
to whether the patient is a vegetarian rather than age. If the treatment
worked well for vegetarians (irrespective of age) but was harmful for meat
eaters, and the 90 year old was a vegetarian while the 60 year old was a
meat eater, then the treatment would be unlikely to work in the 61 year
old and likely to work in the 90 year old. Without specifying high-quality
mechanistic reasoning, we must acknowledge that the underlying mechanisms might be far more complex and uncertain than we believe.

Then, even if we understood all the relevant mechanisms operating in
the participants within a study, those mechanisms must be stable between
study and routine practice populations in order to be useful for generalizing. The belief that mechanisms are stable is widely held amongst philosophers of science. Consider some excerpts from the recent literature:

> . . .entities and activities organized such that they are productive of
> *regular* changes from start or set-up to finish or termination condi-
> tions [401].

> . . .the existence of a mechanism provides evidence of the stability of a
> causal relationship. If we can single out a plausible mechanism, then
> that mechanism is likely to occur in a range of individuals, making
> the causal relation stable over a variety of populations [403].

> Nomological machines [mechanisms] generate causal laws between
> inputs and predictable outputs [53].

The belief that biochemical mechanisms are stable might be borrowed from
physics where, if we ignore the quantum level, there are many engines
that are productive of stable input–output relationships. For instance, Cartwright cites the example of toasters as mechanisms [54]. Nobody would
deny that a toaster's mechanism is useful for predicting whether or not
the bread will get toasted. But mechanisms in the human body and social
world, especially those that are pertinent to clinically relevant outcomes,
are generally far more complex than toasters, and might be so sensitive to
initial conditions (or downright unstable) that they could be close to useless for generalizing.

To illustrate the problem with unstable biochemical/psychological mechanisms, reconsider the CCTV example Cartwright uses. Presumably the
mechanism for CCTV effects would be gathered within an empirical study
of thieves and why they choose not to steal cars under certain circumstances. Say that such a study revealed that the thieves in the study were

extremely scared of getting caught, but that they were not deterred by the visibility of the cameras. CCTV cameras would stop these thieves by promoting vigilance, while high visibility of the CCTV cameras might not be as important. But there is no reason to assume that the mechanism (fear of getting caught) was stable across populations of thieves.

There is another reason to doubt the stability of mechanisms. Most mechanisms are discovered in tightly controlled laboratory experiments – often in animal models (exposing the link between ethics and methodology once again) – that expressly ignore as many potentially interfering variables as possible. Why should we accept supposed causes discovered in tightly controlled laboratory systems more than we believe in supposed causes discovered in (tightly controlled) randomized trials? The paradoxical drug responses cited earlier are counterexamples to the view that causal pathways discovered in one setting are generalizable.

10.6.2 The problem with using mechanism-based subgroup analysis to generalize the results of studies

Another supposed solution to the problem of generalizability is to employ subgroup analysis. Here we examine not only the average response, but also the response in various subgroups (such as smokers, the elderly, or women). If we could isolate subgroups that were responders (or in whom the treatment harmed), then we would be able to predict whether an individual was likely to benefit or be harmed by a treatment. There are many problems with subgroup analysis that are beyond the scope of this work to discuss in detail. I will limit myself here to describing perhaps the most serious problem and explaining why mechanisms are neither necessary nor sufficient to solve it.

The basic problem with subgroup analysis is that if we identify a sufficient number of subgroups, some of them will appear to respond significantly differently from the average due to chance alone. If, for example, we use classical hypothesis tests with 0.05 as our significance level to measure potential differences between subgroups and the average, we would expect 1 out of 20 subgroups to display significant differences due to chance alone. The authors of the Second International Study of Infarct Survival (ISIS-2) illustrate the problem in an amusing way:

> When in a trial with a clearly positive overall result many subgroup analyses are considered, *false negative* results in some particular subgroups must be expected [and vice versa]. For example, subdivision of the patients in ISIS-2 with respect to their astrological birth signs appears to indicate that for patients born under Gemini or Libra

there was a slightly adverse effect of aspirin on mortality (9% SD 13 increase; NS), while for patients born under all other astrological signs there was a strikingly beneficial effect (28% SD 5 reduction; $2p < 0.00001$) [468].

Supporters of mechanisms such as La Caze claim that the problem with spurious subgroup analysis disappears when the subgroups are based on mechanisms.

The problem with La Caze's solution is that he fails to appreciate that fertile imaginations can think of plausible mechanisms for just about anything. A mechanism for retroactive prayer [469] has even been described. La Caze would no doubt respond that the mechanism for retroactive prayer was not based on a truly plausible mechanism. But unless he distinguishes between high- and low-quality mechanisms (which he does not), he cannot dismiss the mechanism for retroactive prayer without exposing himself to the objection that he would also have suppressed Semmelweis-type examples. Just as mechanisms can be dreamed up to explain anything, so different mechanism-based subgroups can be dreamed up to explain why any subgroup in a trial responded differently from the average. In short, mechanisms *per se* are not sufficient to overcome the problem with spurious subgroup selection.

Knowledge of mechanisms are also unnecessary for adequate subgroup analysis. Consider the following example. A new drug for terminal cancer is invented that proves, for some unknown reason, to dramatically and completely cure all natural redheads but which has no effect whatsoever on anyone else. Not having a plausible mechanism for why this should be the case would not be a good reason to withhold the drug from redheads. Here we have a legitimate subgroup but no plausible mechanism. This suggests that mechanisms are unnecessary for identifying subgroups.

10.6.3 Mechanisms are not the only game in town when it comes to generating hypotheses

In the public imagination antibiotics came to symbolize the almost limitless possibilities of science. Yet this is not entirely merited, for, as will be seen, the discovery of penicillin was not the product of scientific reasoning but rather an accident – much more improbable than is commonly appreciated.

—J. LeFanu [94]

Hypotheses about treatment effects are (often) based on sound mechanistic reasoning. A celebrated example of a mechanism-generated hypothesis was Louis Pasteur's use of the germ theory of disease to explain the causes of many ailments and their prevention by vaccination. For example, it is difficult to see how Pasteur's idea for a rabies vaccine would have arisen without the germ theory.

We would expect that these treatments are more likely to have positive effects than, say, randomly generated treatments. Given that mechanism-generated hypotheses are more likely to be confirmed than randomly generated hypotheses, it seems reasonable to conclude that mechanisms provide some degree of confirmatory power. In Bayesian terms, they raise the prior probability of the hypothesis.

In response, it is true that mechanisms adds evidential weight (proportional to its quality). However, comparing mechanistically generated hypotheses with randomly generated hypotheses does not support the view that mechanisms are the only or indeed the most efficient way to generate hypotheses. The contrast class is not randomly generated hypotheses, but (perhaps among other things) "observationally" derived hypotheses. There are currently many treatments that are widely believed to work on (admittedly weak) empirical grounds yet have not been adequately tested. For example, there is a considerable body of anecdotal and observational evidence dating back to Babylonian times that chicken soup has therapeutic benefits, especially for colds and flu [470]. Despite a lack of high-quality comparative clinical research, many people believe that chicken soup is effective and use it. One could view the extensive anecdotal and observational evidence as a hypothesis worth testing more rigorously. Remedies ranging from gargling with salt water to cure sore throats to eating hot (spicy) foods to cure the common cold are supported by a large volume of anecdotal evidence.

Rigorously testing these observationally generated hypotheses in high-quality comparative research would also serve a very useful practical benefit over testing hypotheses generated by the basic sciences. Basic science usually yields hypotheses about therapies that are not currently in use. If the hypothesis derived from laboratory research is confirmed, then the therapy might benefit people. However, if it turns out that the therapy under examination is useless or harmful, nobody would be helped. The situation is quite different when we test whether existent therapies are effective or harmful. If it turns out that they are effective, then, like therapies derived from mechanistic research, they could benefit people by leading to more widespread use. But even if the therapy proved harmful in a trial, then the knowledge could benefit people by discouraging its use.

We might be tempted to believe that chicken soup-type treatments are less likely to prove effective than artificially engineered therapies developed in the laboratory. This may not be the case. A recent study of hypotheses generated by basic science research warns us how rare they are. The study examined 101 "mechanistic" findings that claimed to have a clinically relevant implication in top basic science journals (*Science, Nature, Cell, Journal of Experimental Medicine, Journal of Clinical Investigation,* and *Journal of Biological Chemistry*) between 1979 and 1983 [471]. Twenty years later, in 2002, 27 of the allegedly promising technologies had been tested in comparative clinical studies, 19 indicated a "positive" (statistically significant) benefit of the technology, and five had been approved for marketing. One can only assume that the reason the remaining 14 were not approved for marketing was that they were dangerous or were impractical (i.e. too expensive). Of the five approved for marketing, only one has what the authors of the study claim is a clinically relevant outcome. In short, of "positive" mechanistic findings (those which appear to have a clinically relevant benefit), only 5% turn out to have some benefit, and even fewer (1% in this study) seem to have clinically relevant effects.

It is fair to assume that if this study were expanded to include the top 20 or 100 basic science journals, the proportion of clinical breakthroughs would decrease substantially. We should also keep in mind that basic research is an enormously expensive way to generate hypotheses compared with ready-made anecdotal evidence.

10.7 Recommending a (slightly) more important role for mechanistic reasoning in the EBM system

The claim that understanding mechanisms is required for *establishing* that medical interventions produce their putative patient-relevant outcomes is mistaken. On the other hand, refusing any role at all for mechanistic reasoning violates the principle of total evidence. To be sure, EBM proponents are correct to point out the many limits to our knowledge of bodily mechanisms and their interactions. However, not all mechanistic reasoning was created equal. High-quality mechanistic reasoning involves inferences from "not incomplete" mechanisms that take into account the possibility of triggering other mechanisms or of altering the nature of every mechanism being relied on to produce the targeted outcomes. High-quality mechanistic reasoning can bolster the strength of evidence in favor of claims that treatments are effective, and in some exceptional cases suffice to support claims that a medical therapy is effective alone.

If I am correct that high-quality mechanistic reasoning can, and should, be used to support hypotheses that treatments have their putative effects, hierarchies of study designs, should replaced by a system whereby evidence of sufficiently high quality should be *combined*. There are at least two practical ways to combine mechanistic reasoning with evidence from comparative clinical studies. One is to add a further criterion for upgrading evidence in the GRADE system. We would upgrade studies if they were bolstered by high-quality mechanistic reasoning. However, this would not help in cases where there are no comparative clinical studies. Another way would be to consider high-quality mechanistic reasoning as a separate potential source of evidence (see Figure 10.5). Here, hypotheses supported by both high-quality comparative clinical studies mechanistic reasoning would be deemed more strongly supported by evidence than hypotheses supported by one form of evidence alone.

Appendix: cases where mechanistic reasoning led to the adoption of therapies that were either useless or harmful according to well-conducted clinical research

Table 10.1 Cases where mechanistic reasoning suggested a treatment had a positive effect for a particular disorder and comparative clinical studies (not necessarily randomized trials) suggested that the treatment had a negative effect for the same disorder

Ailment	Conclusion based on mechanistic reasoning	Conclusion based on comparative studies
Sudden cardiac death	Arrhythmias lead to sudden cardiac death. Antiarrhythmic drugs will reduce arrhythmias and hence reduce mortality due do sudden cardiac death	Antiarrhythmic drugs increase mortality due to sudden cardiac death [112,113]
Sudden infant death syndrome (SIDS)	Placing babies to sleep on their stomachs will reduce mortality from SIDS [472]	Placing babies to sleep on their backs cuts mortality from SIDS in half [428]
Human growth hormone (HGH) for hypercatabolism (breakdown of body tissue)	HGH builds body tissue and will therefore reduce the rate of hypercatabolism	HGH increases morbidity and mortality [351]

(Continued)

Table 10.1 (Continued)

Ailment	Conclusion based on mechanistic reasoning	Conclusion based on comparative studies
Organ failure	A cause of oxygen failure is reduced oxygen. Therefore, increasing oxygen delivery will cure organ failure	Increased oxygen delivery is detrimental to organs [352,353]
Menopausal symptoms including increased risk of cardiac disease	Reduced levels of hormones cause menopausal symptoms. Therefore, hormone replacement therapy (HRT) will reduce menopausal symptoms	HRT has a detrimental effect on menopausal symptoms including cardiac disease [209]
Breast cancer	Breast cancer is "local." Therefore radical mastectomy will remove cancer and improve chances of recovery from breast cancer [473]	Radical mastectomy for breast cancer is associated with higher mortality than lumpectomy and radiation [24,138,139]
Recovery from trauma	Rest will improve recovery rate	Rest sometimes leads to increased recovery time [24,474]
Early screening for breast cancer	Early screening for breast cancer leads to early diagnosis, early treatment, and better outcomes	Early screening for breast cancer has no positive effect, and possibly a mild harmful effect [211,475,476]

Table 10.2 Cases where mechanistic reasoning suggested a treatment had a positive effect for a particular disorder and comparative clinical studies (not necessarily randomized trials) suggested that the treatment had no effect on the same disorder but might have had harmful side-effects

Ailment	Mechanistic reasoning	Comparative studies
Brain damage after stroke	Nimodipine reduces risk of brain damage after stroke	Nimodipine has no positive effect [24]
Eczema	Evening primrose oil cures eczema (because eczema was allegedly caused by the body's failure to metabolize γ-linolenic acid, or GLA, and evening primrose oil contains GLA)	Evening primrose oil has no effect [477,478]
Septic shock (caused by infection and leads to dangerously low blood pressure and organ failure)	Gram-negative bacteria cause septic shock by releasing endotoxins into the bloodstream, which stimulate cells to release cytokines. Cytokines damage	The antibodies turned out to have a mild negative effect [24]

Table 10.2 (Continued)

Ailment	Mechanistic reasoning	Comparative studies
	blood vessels, causing blood to leak and subsequent drop in blood pressure and shock. Antibodies that neutralized the cytokines will therefore raise blood pressure to normal levels	
Early screening in general for prevention	Early screening will lead to early detection and the possibility for more efficient treatment (whereas late detection often means that the disease is too severe to treat)	There is little evidence that early screening is beneficial [24]
Regular dental check-ups	Regular dental check-ups screen for problems that, if detected early, can be better cured	There is no evidence for the benefit of regular dental check-ups [24]
Impacted wisdom teeth	Removing healthy impacted wisdom teeth prevents future damage	Removing healthy impacted wisdom teeth has no positive effect on the target outcome, and causes harmful side-effects from surgery [479]
Circulatory support for patients with trauma	Medical anti-shock trousers will increase venous return to the heart until definitive care can be given	Evidence suggests no benefit of medical anti-shock trousers [480]
Prostatic hypertrophy	Finasteride inhibits a hormone responsible for enlarging the prostate and will therefore cure the hypertrophy	Finasteride and terazosin have no positive effect on prostatic hypertrophy [481]
Osteoarthritis of the knee	Osteoarthritis of the knee is often caused by meniscus, ligament, or cartilage damage. These can be cured by arthroscopic surgery	Arthroscopic surgery for osteoarthritis of the knee has no benefit [276]
Heart disease	Laboratory experiments suggest that vitamin E reduces the risk of coronary heart disease and atherosclerosis	Vitamin E has no positive impact on heart disease and atherosclerosis [204]
Fracture prevention in postmenopausal women	Fluoride salts are capable of increasing bone density, therefore fluoride salts will reduce the incidence of fractures	Sodium fluoride does not reduce fracture incidence [482]
Neuroblastoma (a rare malignant tumor affecting young children)	Children diagnosed before the age of 1 have a better outlook, therefore implement a screening technique (using urine)	The screening had no benefit for the target disorder, but the harms included unjustified surgery and chemotherapy [483]

Table 10.3 Cases where failure to provide a mechanism delayed the acceptance of therapies that appeared, based on comparative clinical studies, to be effective

Ailment	Mechanistic reasoning	Comparative clinical study
Puerperal fever	Semmelweis failed to provide a mechanism for how washing hands with chlorinated lime might prevent puerperal fever	Semmelweis introduced hand-washing and reduced the rates of puerperal fever [484], but his suggestion was not adopted until the germ theory of disease became accepted after his death [89]
Peptic ulcer	It was believed that bacteria could not live in the stomach wall and therefore that bacteria could not cause peptic ulcers	Marshall dramatically swallowed *Helicobacter pylori* bacteria, developed an ulcer, and cured himself with antibiotics [485,486]
Eclampsia (seizures during pregnancy)	The mechanism of action of magnesium for eclampsia was unknown, and many doctors, especially in the UK, refused to use it despite evidence from many comparative clinical studies	A large-scale randomized trial reported in *The Lancet* [487] finally persuaded the medical community

Knowledge *that* versus knowledge *how*: situating the EBM position on expert clinical judgment

There is a suspicion that the judgments of clinicians would be more reliable if rendered more rational by following explicit rules and recipes for diagnosis and treatment. …Yet others would see in clinical judgment, decisions made on the basis of an intuition born of years of bedside experience, and not reducible to explicit formulae.

—H.T.J. Englehardt [488]

…it is easy to move from holding that scientifically tested beliefs are more authoritative to holding that scientists themselves should have more authority than non-scientists when it comes to assessing knowledge, claims, or proposals.

—B. Djulbegovic, G.H. Guyatt & R.E. Ashcroft [4]

11.1 Controversies surrounding the EBM stance on expert clinical judgement

The view that experts have special access to knowledge goes back at least as far as Plato [489]. In medicine this view has been particularly influential: experienced clinicians are often believed to possess tacit knowledge and intuition that cannot be reduced to mechanical rules. The deference to expert judgment is also reflected in the way doctors are trained. After

The Philosophy of Evidence-Based Medicine, First Edition. Jeremy Howick.
© 2011 Jeremy Howick. Published 2011 by Blackwell Publishing Ltd.

spending 2–3 years studying basic sciences, medical students spend the next 2–3 years doing clinical work, where they serve as apprentices to more senior (expert) colleagues in hospital. Indeed, if we did not trust that our doctors knew what is best for us, we would not allow them to prod, prick, or cut us and we would not accept their prescriptions for powerful pharmacological drugs, many of which have known deleterious effects.

In fact, until very recently, expert judgments were deemed to be the ultimate authority on the safety and efficacy of medical interventions. An NIH report in the USA, published in 1990, opened with the following words:

> Group judgment methods are perhaps the most widely used means of assessment of medical technologies in many countries. The consensus development conference is a relatively inexpensive and rapid mechanism for the consideration and evaluation of different attributes of a medical technology including, for example, safety, efficacy, and efficiency, among many others [103].

The report was also supported by official representatives from Canada [104], Denmark [105], Finland [106], the Netherlands [107], Norway [108], Sweden [109], and the UK [110].

Experts on the consensus panel were supposed to review the available evidence [490]. However, the connection between the consensus statement and the best available evidence was often spurious. There was no requirement that the evidence should come from clinical research. It should not be surprising, therefore, that the expert judgments were often at odds with results from comparative clinical studies. In fact, one of the members of the consensus panel complained about the disparity between available randomized trials and expert consensus in his contribution on page 29 of the NIH report [490]. Other studies have highlighted the difference between expert opinion and the results of conclusive comparative clinical studies. For instance, Antman *et al.* [111] found that textbook recommendations for treatments intended for heart attack routinely

> ...failed to mention important advances or exhibited delays in recommending effective preventive measures. In some cases, treatments that have no effect on mortality or are potentially harmful continued to be recommended by several clinical experts.

Trish Greenhalgh amusingly describes the method of expert consensus as the GOBSAT ("Good Old Boys Sat Around the Table") method [257].

Against this backdrop, we saw in chapter 2 that EBM proponents advocate the epistemic superiority of comparative clinical research, especially
researching stemming from systematic reviews of randomized trials. The
EBM position on evidence is most clearly expressed in the various "hierarchies" of evidence. Although there are many different hierarchies, they
all share the property of either not including expert judgment at all [19]
or placing it at the very bottom of the list [21]. To be fair, EBM proponents
have insisted on the importance of expertise as a tool when used alongside
research evidence [12,32], but rarely allow expert judgment as an admissible type of evidence.

In fact, Dave Sackett, a founder of the EBM movement, believes that
all experts should retire as soon as they reach the status of expert. In a
paper entitled "The Sins of Expertise and a proposal for redemption," he
writes:

> ...experts...commit two sins that retard the advance of science...
> Firstly, adding our prestige to our opinions gives the latter far greater
> persuasive power than they deserve...The second sin...is committed
> on grant applications and manuscripts that challenge current expert
> consensus...in 1983 I wrote a paper calling for the compulsory retire-
> ment of experts and never again lectured, wrote, or refereed anything
> to do with compliance [33].

Sackett takes his own medicine; he stopped discussing EBM in 2000.

As it stands there are two problems with the EBM position on expertise.
First, it is ambiguous. There are several distinct roles for expertise/expert
judgment, including the following.

1 The clinical judgment that a therapy has its putative effects on average
(I shall call this *general clinical judgment*).
2 The clinical judgment that a therapy is effective for an individual (I shall
call this *individual clinical judgment*).
3 A clinical judgment about how the best evidence can be integrated with
patient values and circumstances (I shall call this *integrating expertise*).
4 An agent that potentially amplifies the therapeutic benefit of an intervention, perhaps by enhancing placebo effects (I shall call this *therapeutic expertise*).
5 As an agent that performs various tasks involved in the clinical encounter, such as recognizing symptoms, elucidating signs, taking blood
pressure, or performing a surgical operation (I shall call this *clinical
expertise*).

Broadly speaking, the first two roles for clinical judgment involve generating evidence, while the last three involve tacit knowledge [491].

The second problem with the EBM position has to do with the placement of expert judgment in the EBM hierarchy. The view that comparative clinical studies (such as randomized trials) belong *above* (or have any hierarchical relation to) expert judgment is not supported by sustained arguments.

In this chapter I will address both problems by demonstrating that although the EBM position on expert judgment *as evidence* is well supported by a plethora of largely ignored studies, other roles for expert judgment are important and they deserve more discussion within the EBM literature.

11.2 General clinical judgment belongs at the bottom of (or off) the hierarchy of evidence

Established practices are difficult to challenge without causing concern amongst those who have helped to establish them. By the time they are established they are firmly believed to serve the patient's interests and therefore it is not an easy matter to walk in from the comfort of an epidemiology unit and start suggesting withholding them from some individuals because you want to apply something called a randomised controlled trial.

—A. Cochrane & M. Blythe [492]

A celebrated example of the GOBSAT method at work is represented by the Cochrane Collaboration logo (Figure 11.1). The horizontal lines in the logo represent a series of trials that tested the benefits of a short inexpensive course of corticosteroids for women who were ready to give birth prematurely. Of interest are the data related to infant mortality due to complications of immaturity. Horizontal lines touching the vertical line indicate no clear benefit of the drug. Horizontal lines lying to the left of the vertical line indicate that the drug had a positive benefit. A smaller horizontal line indicates that the result is more precise. The diamond represents the combined effect of the treatment in all of the studies.

The first trial (represented by the lowest horizontal line) was conducted in 1972 and did not find a positive benefit for the drug. Many further smaller trials were conducted over the next two decades, but their results were inconsistent. Some found a mild benefit, while others found none. In 1981, Patricia Crowley reviewed the existing evidence systematically [116]. She located four randomized trials of sufficiently high quality [117–120]. Combined, those studies observed approximately 1000 infants who received antenatal steroids and a similar number of infants who received placebos. Of those who received antenatal steroids, 70 died, while 130 in the placebo group died. The difference was statistically significant and, given that the outcome was infant mortality, it was clinically relevant as well.

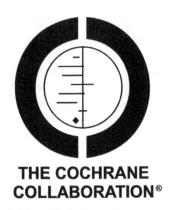

**THE COCHRANE
COLLABORATION®**

Figure 11.1 The Cochrane Collaboration logo.

To Crowley's surprise, the use of corticosteroids did not become routine practice after she published her findings. In 1989 she updated her review to include more trials. The new results were made freely available on the Oxford Database of Perinatal Trials, in the book *Effective Care in Pregnancy and Childbirth* [493] and in a journal article [494]. Still, use of the treatment rarely rose above 20%.

In seeming ignorance of this evidence, trials that involved allocating people to receive placebos rather than steroids continued. It is unlikely that any pregnant woman would have agreed to enter a randomized trial (and risk getting a placebo) after 1981 had they known about the existing evidence. It was only in 1994, when the NIH finally issued a consensus statement in the *Journal of the American Medical Association* [495] that antenatal steroid use became routine practice.

The Cochrane example highlights several problems in medical research including the failure to conduct systematic reviews, the unethical nature of conducting research when convincing results are already known, and the need to get evidence into practice. My purpose here is to illustrate the danger of allowing expert judgment a prominent *evidential* role when solid evidence already exists.

While many experts may have been unaware of the evidence for antenatal steroid use others appealed to their own eminence as a means of disregarding it. Professor Jane Harding, for example, recalls the following:

> ...particularly in the UK, they felt, "Nothing good could come from the colonies" [Crowley was from New Zealand] and the fact of where the trial was done was very relevant. The other thing that they both

said to me was they felt that in many places the paediatricians were the people who were discouraging use, since they felt that they could manage lung disease, that there was not really a problem, and that the obstetricians were treading on their territories, or at least on their toes [496].

Corroborating Harding's experience, John Williams recalls a similar story related to his own reasons for not using corticosteroids in spite of the evidence suggesting that it was helpful.

I am a humble obstetrician, who is a recipient of the literature rather than a contributor, but I was developing during the era of these publications, and here are some of the things that struck me. The first was an oration by Sir Stanley Clayton [President of the Royal College of Obstetricians and Gynaecologists, 1972–75] in 1975 at the American Congress of Obstetricians and Gynecologists, where he said that in his experience as the editor of the grey journal, the *Commonwealth Journal* as it was then, how much rubbish was submitted for publication. He wished that registrars didn't have to do research to get jobs, and it was time it was all stopped. That was the first thing that hit me. And I was then at a meeting in Cardiff where Cliff Roberton spoke, and he seemed to be of the opinion that obstetricians shouldn't be treading on the toes of paediatricians, and that they were very good at looking after babies and we didn't need to interfere. He went on to pour scorn on quite a lot of the uncontrolled and poor publications, and again this struck me. I said, "Why were these published if they were such bad studies?" He replied, "You know, people having a glass of whisky and refereeing a paper, if it's somebody they know they will put it in, if it's not they won't." He was fairly scornful of the poor quality publications, and it gave the impression, certainly in Cardiff, that we shouldn't be using steroids. And that set me back a little way [496].

In another example, Archie Cochrane (who inspired the creation of the Cochrane Collaboration) explained what happened when he reported the preliminary results of a trial that compared home versus hospital treatment for varicose veins. The Medical Research Council gave its ethical approval, but cardiologists in the planned location of the trial (Cardiff) refused to take part because they were certain, based on their expertise, that hospital treatment was far superior. Cochrane reports this great disappointment: "They [the cardiologists]...still felt a sacred right to treat patients as they wished" [492].

Eventually Cochrane succeeded at beginning the trial in Bristol. Six months into the trial, the ethics committee called on Cochrane to compile and report on the preliminary results. At that stage home care showed a slight but not statistically significant benefit. Cochrane, however, decided to play a trick on his colleagues: he prepared two reports, one with the actual number of deaths, and one with the number reversed. The rest of the story is best told from Cochrane's perspective:

> As we were going into the committee, in the anteroom, I showed some cardiologists the results. They were vociferous in their abuse: "Archie," they said, "we always thought you were unethical. You must stop the trial at once." I let them have their way for some time and then apologised and gave them the true results, challenging them to say, as vehemently, that coronary care units should be stopped immediately. There was dead silence and I felt rather sick because they were, after all, my medical colleagues [492].

Anecdotal examples do not, by themselves, support the reliability of clinical expertise relative to comparative clinical studies, not least because such a conclusion would be viciously circular. However, there are additional reasons to believe that experts are not good judges of therapeutic effects of medical interventions. In the rest of this section I will review these empirical and theoretical arguments.

11.2.1 Why mechanical rules outperform clinical judges

The patient, treated on the fashionable theory, sometimes gets well in spite of the medicine. The medicine therefore restored him, and the young doctor received new courage to proceed in his bold experiments on the lives of his fellow creatures.

—Thomas Jefferson [497]

Clinical experience does not provide an adequate basis for detecting modest beneficial or adverse effects. In the Cochrane example cited above there were 130 deaths out of 1000 in the placebo group and 70 deaths out of 1000 in the group taking the drug. Even the busiest obstetrician might only see a few hundred cases per year and would be unlikely to observe any difference whether or not they administered steroids. Unaided by comparative studies, even the best clinical judges will not be able to detect modest effects.

Clinicians can be deceived even in dramatic instances due to the natural course of illness and the placebo effect. In an age of modern medicine it is easy to forget that even serious ailments often go away without any treatment at all. Archie Cochrane tells the following story about his experience as the only physician in a prisoner of war camp in a Dulag (POW transit camp) in the Second World War.

> I was usually the senior medical officer and for a considerable time the only officer and the only doctor. (It was bad enough being a POW, but having me as your doctor was a bit too much.) There were about 20,000 POWs in the camp, of whom a quarter were British. The diet was about 600 calories a day and we all had diarrhoea. In addition we had severe epidemics of typhoid, diphtheria, infections, jaundice, and sand-fly fever, with more than 300 cases of "pitting oedema above the knee." To cope with this we had a ramshackle hospital, some aspirin, some antacid, and some skin antiseptic.
>
> The only real assets were some devoted orderlies, mainly from the Friends' Field Ambulance Unit. Under the best conditions one would have expected an appreciable mortality; there in the Dulag I expected hundreds to die of diphtheria alone in the absence of specific therapy. In point of fact there were only four deaths, of which three were due to gunshot wounds inflicted by the Germans. This excellent result had, of course, nothing to do with the therapy they received or my clinical skill. It demonstrated, on the other hand, very clearly the relative unimportance of therapy in comparison with the recuperative power of the human body. On one occasion, when I was the only doctor there, I asked the German Stabsarzt for more doctors to help me cope with these fantastic problems. He replied: "Nein! Aerzte sind ueberfluessig." ("No! Doctors are superfluous.") I was furious and even wrote a poem about it; later I wondered if he was wise or cruel; he was certainly right [498].

Of course the POWs in Cochrane's story are unrepresentative in that they were young and, at the time of their recruitment, healthier than average. On the other hand, their injuries, illnesses, poor diet, and lack of morale may have compensated for these benefits. There are many other examples where natural history of illness has confused even the most astute clinicians. The radical Halsted mastectomy (named after its American inventor William Stewart Halsted) is tragic example of how clinicians can mistake natural history with treatment benefits. The radical mastectomies sometimes left women with nothing other than a thin layer of skin covering their heart. Surgeons noted that many of their patients died soon after the mutilating operations. Even the earliest (1898) studies noted almost a 50% mortality rate 3 years after the operation [473], yet the procedure continued to be common for almost a century in the USA [138]. Faced with these statistics, surgeons no doubt supposed that had these women not undergone the radical and disfiguring surgery, even more would have died. By the 1980s well-conducted long-term studies demonstrated convincingly that minor surgery (lumpectomy) combined with radiation and sometimes chemotherapy were as effective as Halsted mastectomy, and far less damaging to the woman's body [24,139,499]. It is also interesting that the surgical procedure might have remained popular in the USA long after it had been abandoned elsewhere because William Stewart Halsted was a revered expert and national hero [138].

Placebo effects can sometimes exacerbate the confusion between real treatment effects and natural history. A clinician might observe dramatic remission from depression after Prozac therapy, but without further investigation it is impossible to conclude that the recovery was due to the characteristic feature of the treatment (fluoxetine hydrochloride), spontaneous resolution, or placebo effects. Empirical studies have shown that patients report superior outcomes when they believe they are receiving a brand name [500], expensive [501], and powerful [262,502] drug that is delivered by a sympathetic physician [258]. These potentially beneficial features of a treatment process can easily confuse even the most astute clinician. To make things worse, the clinician's belief can itself enhance the effects of the treatment and vice versa [405]. Unaided by careful comparative clinical studies, clinicians will not always be able to distinguish between natural history and placebo effects.

The limits to detection of large and small effects are exacerbated by the common reasoning fallacies of naive and well-educated clinicians (and most other people). These fallacies are well documented and they include ignoring base-rates and sample sizes, misperceiving chance, engaging in the gambler's fallacy, using the law of small numbers, disregarding predictability, and disregarding regression to the mean and others [503,504].

To sum up, experience alone is usually an insufficient tool for detecting small and large effects. Hence, the EBM movement is correct to place clinical expertise (as *general clinical judgment*) at the bottom of the hierarchy (Figure 11.2). Where high-quality comparative clinical trials do exist, data should trump the judgment of experts in diagnostic, prognostic, and therapeutic predictions.

Many clinicians will be prepared to admit that as far as average predictions about a group go, well controlled studies are superior to clinical judgment. However, those same clinicians might still insist that clinical judgment is required to apply the average results to an individual patient. As Mant states: "The paradox of the clinical trial is that it is the best way to

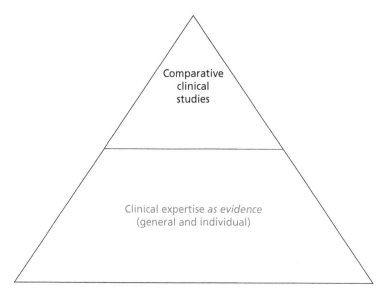

Figure 11.2 The correct place for expert judgment in a simplified EBM hierarchy.

assess whether an intervention works, but it is arguably the worst way to assess who will benefit from it" [62].

In the next section I will consider the role of *individual* expert clinical judgment.

11.3 Individual clinical judgment also belongs at the bottom of the hierarchy

[A]pplied science, engineering for example, has never felt that constructing a single bridge presents any conceptual difficulties for the application of general knowledge. Science, applied in practice, does not cease to be science, nor do the methods of making such application seem to involve any fundamental departure from scientific conceptions of hypothesis and confirmation.

—E. Sober [505]

Far, therefore, from arguing that the statistical approach is impossible in the fact of human variability, we must realise that it is because of variability that it is essential.

—A.B. Hill & I.D. Hill [2]

Applying average trial results to individuals is problematic. Say there are 1000 people in a trial of a new antidepressant and 500 of those people recover completely, while the other 500 do not experience any benefit whatsoever. The average outcome of this study is that the antidepressant leads to a 50% recovery rate even though none of the patients in the trial experienced a 50% recovery. As Peter Rothwell points out, "[a] single patient cannot experience a 50% reduction in death or a 20% improvement in survival" [506]. The average results of this trial would not tell us what would happen to an individual patient. An exception might arise if researchers were to identify a characteristic that makes a particular patient a responder. Outside pharmacogenetics, this solution is rarely as simple as it sounds, largely due to the problems associated with subgroup analysis, as discussed in the previous chapter. More importantly, once we have identified a subgroup of responders, the problem of applying average results *of that subgroup* to an individual within the subgroup crops up again.

However potential problems with applying average trial results to individuals does not imply that expert judgment can improve matters. In fact, a preponderance of evidence I will consider in some detail below suggests otherwise.

> An advocate of this anti-actuarial position would have to maintain, for the sake of logical consistency, that if one is forced to play Russian roulette a single time and is allowed to select a gun with one or five bullets in a chamber, the uniqueness of the event makes the choice arbitrary [507].

The hypothesis that expert judgment is useful in applying average statistical results to individual patients has been tested hundreds of times over the course of the last six decades. With a mere handful of exceptions, they all suggest that following "mechanical" rules is as good as, or better than, expert judgment (even when the experts have access to the same data that generated the mechanical rule). In the next section I will review this evidence.

11.3.1 Empirical data supporting the view that mechanical rule-following is superior to expert clinical judgment

...we are treating the possibility of gold in the brains of clinicians as if it is not worth mining, or so obviously present that it is not worth investigation, and neither situation has any support. This attitude is affecting our thinking, our training, our research and our practice and it's killing people as well as under- or over-rating clinicians.

—M. Scriven [508]

In 1954 Paul Meehl conducted a systematic review of studies comparing predictions based on expert judgment with predictions based on following mechanical rules. To Meehl, the "mechanical" method involved a prediction arrived at by some straightforward application of an equation or table to the data [509]. Provided that the clinician did not explicitly follow a mechanical rule, Meehl categorized the clinician's strategy as "nonmechanical" or "informal." Overall, Meehl reviewed 20 studies comparing the predictive accuracy of expert judges compared with mechanical rulefollowing, and found that only one study contradicted the observed trend, suggesting the superiority of clinical over mechanical prediction. In the remaining studies, mechanical rules were as good as, or better than, clinical judgment.

In a subsequent typical study, expert clinical judgments were compared with mechanical diagnoses of abdominal pain in 304 patients. The study addressed whether a computer (following mechanical rules) or an expert clinician (with access to the same data as the computer) more accurately diagnosed patients who had been admitted to hospital with abdominal pain. For example, the two methods predicted whether the patient had acute appendicitis. Subsequent surgery then verified the accuracy of the diagnosis. Overall, the computer diagnosis was over 10% more accurate than expert diagnosis (91.8% vs. 79.6%). The computer accurately predicted acute appendicitis requiring immediate surgery in 99% of cases, whereas expert clinicians only diagnosed acute appendicitis in 88% of cases [510].

In the 25 years succeeding Meehl's original publication, several reviews replicated Meehl's original study [511–515]. One study even showed that linear equations with randomly assigned coefficients can generate correct diagnoses better than expert judges [513]. In addition, the exception reported by Meehl did not survive replication. Hence, when Scriven reported on Meehl's thesis in 1977 he stated: "there are at the moment…no cases in which any *group* of experts has been able to outperform a formula, where enough study has been done to make it possible to construct a formula" [508].

However, Holt [516,517] pointed out two important flaws in the design of the surveys, namely (i) many of the studies chosen were too small, and (ii) the studies were chosen selectively to support the conclusion that actuarial prediction is superior to clinical prediction. Yet even Holt did not doubt that his objections would overturn Meehl's overall conclusion [517].

Recently, Grove *et al.* [514] took Holt's objections into account and conducted an extensive systematic review that excluded poorly conducted studies. The authors identified all studies within psychology and medicine, where at least one human judge was compared with one mechanical prediction scheme, and where both the judges and mechanical procedures had access to the same data about the predictor variables. They excluded studies predicting non-human outcomes (such as the results of horse races) and studies where the clinical judges and mechanical procedures operated on different sets of participants (unless the assignment to groups was random). They identified 136 studies (51 of which were medical) that met their inclusion criteria, and only eight indicated that clinical judgment was superior. On average, mechanical prediction was 10% more accurate than clinical judgment. Even the eight exceptional studies are what might arise due to chance given the small absolute difference between clinical and mechanical predictive accuracy.

Grove *et al.* searched for, but did not identify, a variable that predicted that clinical judgment would outperform mechanical rules. We might have expected, for example, that the more experienced clinicians performed better. In fact, the opposite seems to be the case. Indeed, a more recent study found an inverse relationship between experience and quality of care [518]. Similarly, time spent with patients did not seem to affect the accuracy of predictions: in studies where clinicians had access to an interview, their predictions were relatively worse [514].

Most clinicians, like most drivers, no doubt believe they are better than average. But by definition most cannot be better than average [519]. Also, the clinicians who outperformed the mechanical rules will no doubt believe that it was their skill rather than chance. To determine whether the clinicians who outperformed the mechanical rule did so by chance, some form of longitudinal study measuring whether a clinician's superiority was replicable would presumably be required. Until such research has been done, the best available empirical research suggests that allowing clinicians to "break" the mechanical rule will tend to make outcomes worse. In Meehl's words,

> ...let me emphasize the brute fact that we have here, depending on one's standards for admission as relevant, from 16 to 20 studies involving a comparison of clinical and actuarial methods, in all but one of which the predictions made actuarially were either approximately equal or superior to those made by a clinician [509].

There are two potentially important differences between comparative clinical studies and mechanical rules. First, very few of the mechanical rules in the Grove meta-analysis involved therapeutic predictions. However, the ones that did compare predictions of therapeutic effects seemed to follow the same trend [520]. However, there were too few studies comparing the accuracy of therapeutic predictions to draw any general conclusions.

It would be interesting to conduct further empirical work in this area. Yet given the consistent trend in favor of mechanical rules for all other types of predictions, one might argue that the burden of proof is on those who claim that therapeutic predictions are the exception.

Second, comparative clinical studies are not the same as mechanical rules. Whereas comparative clinical studies tell us whether, on average, a medical therapy appears to have its putative effects, mechanical rules use statistical tools (often Bayesian analyses) to generate predictions based on a series of variables. For example, a mechanical rule that predicted whether a treatment was likely to work might consider factors such as age, sex, severity of disease, and presence of concomitant medication. Yet the regression analysis that generated the mechanical rule would essentially be a comparative clinical study comparing groups with varying "strengths" of the relevant variables. In short, the difference between mechanical rules as described in the Meehl/Grove studies and comparative clinical studies as I have described them may be trivial. A mechanical rule that predicted therapeutic response could be derived quite straightforwardly from a comparative clinical study.

To sum up, the overwhelming body of evidence suggesting that actuarial judgment is at least as good as clinical judgment has been ignored. Very recently, however, "clinical prediction rules" have gained some traction amongst practitioners. A famous example is the Ottawa ankle rule, which has reduced the number of unnecessary radiographs by 30–40% without increasing the rate of missed fractures at all and saved millions of dollars [521,522]. The Ottawa ankle rule recommends radiography only if there is any pain in the malleolar zone and any one of the following:

1 bone tenderness along the distal 6 cm of the posterior edge of the tibia or tip of the medial malleolus, *or*
2 bone tenderness along the distal 6 cm of the posterior edge of the fibula or tip of the lateral malleolus, *or*
3 an inability to bear weight both immediately and in the emergency department for four steps (Figure 11.3).

Other highly useful clinical prediction rules include the Ottawa knee rules for predicting whether knee radiography is required [523], APACHE II (Acute Physiology and Chronic Health Evaluation) rule for determining severity of patients in intensive care units [524], and many others [525].

To be sure, there are many objections to the view that mechanical rules and comparative clinical studies are superior to expert judgment for predictions about both individual and average therapeutic effects. In conversation, many clinicians object that the evidence supporting the superiority of mechanical rules needs to be examined more carefully. It is true that many studies upon which clinical prediction rules are based have flaws [526].

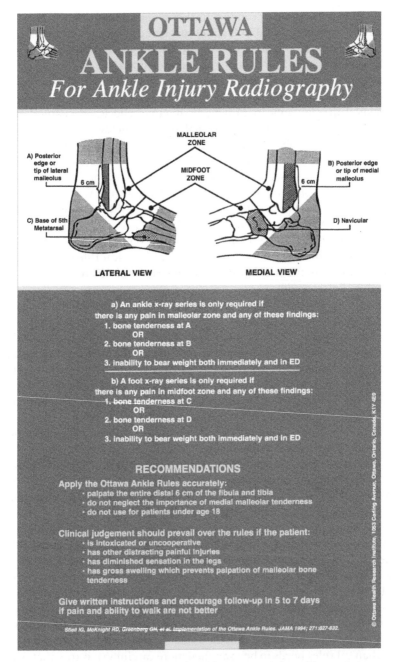

Figure 11.3 The Ottawa ankle rule (reproduced from www.ohri.ca with permission from Ottawa Hospital Research Institute).

But the relevant question is whether, in spite of these flaws, mechanical rules outperform clinical judgment when it comes to evidence that a treatment has its putative effects. In fact, this objection is unacceptable given the large body of diverse studies with such a uniform answer. Writing in 1986, Meehl suggests that the reply to this objection is nothing short of irrational human conduct:

> I would be interested in knowing whether any readers want to controvert the following claim: There is no controversy in social science that shows such a large body of qualitatively diverse studies coming out so uniformly in the same direction as this one. When you are pushing 90 investigations, predicting everything from the outcome of football games to diagnosis of liver disease and when you can hardly come up with a half dozen studies showing even a weak tendency in favour of the clinician, it is time to draw a practical conclusion, whatever theoretical differences may still be disputed. Why, then, is such a strongly and clearly supported empirical generalization not applied in practice...? Not to argue ad hominem but to explain the fact, I think this is just one more of the numerous examples of the ubiquity and recalcitrance of irrationality in the conduct of human affairs [527].

Another common objection is a variation on the claim that average results are not applicable to individuals outside the study. In fact, many of the studies included in the Grove *et al.* meta-analysis applied the mechanical rules to patients who were not included in the population used to derive the rules, and the results were that mechanical rules still outperformed expert judges. Meehl [509] sums up how the problem of external validity does not provide caregivers warrant to disregard mechanical rules:

> If a clinician says "This one is different" or "It's not like the ones in your table," "This time I'm surer," the obvious question is, "Why should we care whether you think this one is different or whether you are surer?" Again, there is only one rational reply to such a question. We have now to study the success frequency of the clinician's guesses when he asserts that he feels this way. If we have already done so, and found him still behind the hit frequency of the table, we would be well advised to ignore him. Always, we might as well face it, the shadow of the statistician hovers in the background; *always* the actuary will have the final word...
>
> In any given instance, we must decide on whom to place our bets; and there is no rational answer to this question *except* in terms

of relative frequencies. If, when the clinician disagrees with the statistics, he tends to be wrong, then, if we put our best *in individual instances* upon him, we will tend to be wrong also.

Yet another objection is that good-quality trials or mechanical rules are often unavailable. The first reply to this objection is that mechanical rules, in the form of guidelines, are available for many common ailments. Yet many clinicians either outright flout the guidelines or claim that their patient is unlike the patients that were considered when the guidelines were designed. But this is just another form of the claim that expert judgment is required to make *individual* clinical judgments, which I have already considered and found wanting.

To be sure, in some cases a caregiver will see a patient with a completely new condition for which the existing mechanical rules might not apply or simply do not exist, in which case he or she will have to use their best judgment. In other cases, guidelines will not be based on sound underlying evidence, in which case caregivers have no choice but to use their best judgment.

Furthermore, the objection that mechanical rules might be unavailable is not an *in principle* objection against the view that mechanical rules, if available, would be superior to clinical judgment. Rather, it is a call to arms to produce more or better guidelines and clinical prediction rules.

The next objection arises from clinicians' anecdotes of cases in which judgment and intuition saved a life. Consider the following true and particularly dramatic example recounted by Trish Greenhalgh.

> It was Saturday morning. I was on call from 8:30 am. I got a call from one of my partners, Dr B, at 5:45 am. He was on holiday 200 miles away but had been called on his mobile phone by Health Call. One of his patients had rung Health Call and *demanded* a visit by Dr B. No other doctor would do. The family had a child with chicken pox. She had been seen the day before by another partner, Dr R, who has 24 years' experience in general practice and is also a clinical assistant in dermatology. She had said it was "definitely chicken pox" and prescribed fluids, analgesia, and calamine. The child had apparently deteriorated and the parents were worried. They had decided that only Dr B would know what to do. Dr B...asked me to go round immediately and examine the child. I was not yet on call and keen to go for my early morning swim before surgery. What should my next move be?
>
> I asked: "How old is the child? [Answer: 15]. Why the $#*! are you so convinced that these guys are not time wasters?"

He said: "For one thing, this family have been on my list for 17 years and they've never asked for anything. For another thing, they go to the most orthodox synagogue in Golders Green. And there's one more thing I don't like about this case. It wasn't the mother who rang, it was the father. In that family, the father *never* does the kids' health."

I didn't go for my swim. I didn't even stop for a bath or breakfast. I drove straight to the house, where all the lights were off. The father, dressed in Orthodox Jewish style complete with long black coat and hat, came out to meet me and apologised that the lights were on a time switch which he could not override. I got a torch out of the car boot. There were 14 relatives in the room, lined up in silence. All the siblings had been woken up and were standing staring at me. On examination by torchlight, the child was conscious and co-operative, and had a typical chicken pox rash. She was post-pubescent and somewhat overweight. Her BP was 90/50 and pulse 100. She was possibly overbreathing (we all were). She said she couldn't get up, or even sit up. On direct questioning, she said, "I just don't feel well. Maybe I'm a bit faint. No, I haven't fainted or blacked out but it's muzzy and I feel quite scared that something's wrong." I examined her respiratory system. She had a respiratory rate of 20 and no focal signs. That was a shame because I was hoping there would be. I found no other physical signs. So I decided to lie about the chest findings. I admitted her to the Coppetts Wood Hospital by blue light ambulance. As I left the room, the father thanked me profusely for saving his daughter's life.

We didn't hear anything for a month, and they got a discharge summary to say the child had had chicken pox with disseminated intravascular coagulation [blood clotting]. The child had initially been admitted to Intensive Care for 5 days. The parents had been told she was lucky to have survived [528].

This is supposed to be a case where the tacit knowledge of the expert, perhaps gained from experience, played a vital role in saving the child's life.

However, it is unclear how this example (or any similar example) bears on the comparison between individual clinical judgment and mechanical prediction. There was no mechanical rule available to Greenhalgh in the example she discusses. Indeed the sensible (and mechanical) course of action in the face of a serious and unexplained symptom is to conduct more tests. A problem might also arise if we were to use Greenhalgh's example to support the more general claim that clinical judgment trumps mechanical rules. Indeed we would have to balance these rhetorically forceful examples with instances when clinical judgment and intuition resulted in *worse* outcomes than mechanical rule-following would have done.

The last objection I will consider is not philosophical but psychological and sociological. If expert judgment is subservient to mechanical rules, then clinicians might fear that they lose some of their authority. In fact, nothing could be further from the truth. Airplane pilots follow very strict protocols and guidelines that result in fewer crashes, yet nobody believes that airline pilots are unskilled and they seem to enjoy quite a high status in society. Likewise, expert clinicians play other vital roles that are as important, if not more important, than predicting whether a particular therapy is likely to have the best outcome. In the rest of this chapter I will outline the other roles for expertise and where they should fit into an expanded EBM system (see Figure 11.2).

11.4 The equally important non-evidential roles of expertise

...it will be apparent that the role of the clinician is undiminished in a system such as the one we have described. Indeed, in many ways it is enhanced. Thus the system is quite incapable of reliable operation unless the clinician first elicits reliable data from the patient – a curiously "old fashioned" re-emphasis on the traditional values of accurate history-taking and careful clinical examination...What the computing system does is to help the clinician in an area where previous studies...have shown him to be relatively weak, namely in the statistical analysis of large volumes of data. In such a case the clinician merely uses the computer to augment his own capabilities and judgment; and indeed there is ample precedent for this. To take one obvious example, the clinician often uses a stethoscope to augment his ability to hear sounds emanating from within a body cavity.

—J.C. Horrocks *et al.* [529]

The biggest challenge to EBM continues to be ensuring that decisions are consistent with patient values and preferences. Helping to resolve this vexing issue represents a key frontier to EBM.

—B. Djulbegovic, G.H. Guyatt & R.E. Ashcroft [4]

Clinical skill and ability to make accurate observations are required at every stage of the clinical encounter and research design. In this section

I will expand upon the EBM view that expert skills are required for non-evidential purposes.

11.4.1 Expert judgment is required to integrate patient values and circumstances with best external evidence

Even the best (statistical or clinical) prediction does not lead straightforwardly to a judgment about the best clinical action. The question of what therapy, if any, the clinician should prescribe is distinct from the question of what the best therapy actually is. Confounding the two constitutes the perennial error of deriving an *ought* from an *is* [388]. To make a sound clinical decision, patient values and circumstances must be integrated with the best therapeutic prediction.

The following imaginary example illustrates this case quite clearly. Imagine an athlete has just advanced to the Olympic rowing final with the best time in the semi-final and is favored to win gold. However, shortly after the semi-final she experiences severe back pain that prevents her from practising or sleeping. Several physicians determine that the main cause of the pain is a sprained ligament. Several randomized trials suggest that the most effective treatment involves ice, ibuprofen, and rest for 3 days. Failure to rest (including doing strenuous exercise), but using ice and ibuprofen, will relieve the pain but delay recovery. Clearly the *most effective* treatment, in a general sense, is not the most appropriate treatment for the star athlete. This example illustrates how the circumstances (the day before the Olympic final) and values (the athlete is willing to delay recovery in order to have a chance of winning a medal) suggest that the most acceptable course of action involves taking what the clinician and patient know well to be the second most effective treatment.

Although, in principle, a machine could integrate therapeutic predictions with patient values and circumstances, it seems unlikely that such a machine will be available in the near future. At present, therefore, a skilled clinician is better placed to integrate these important factors to make a sound clinical decision (Figure 11.4).

Given that expert judgment should not be used as evidence, and that it is important for integrating knowledge of effectiveness with patient values and circumstances, the description of EBM should be changed from "Evidence-based medicine (EBM) requires the integration of the best research evidence with our clinical expertise and our patient's unique values and circumstances" [34] to "EBM requires clinical expertise to integrate the best research evidence with patient values and circumstances."

The new characterization of EBM points to ways in which medical school curricula in general, and EBM textbooks and workshops in particular,

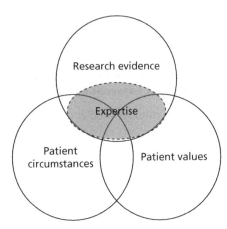

Figure 11.4 Expert judgment plays a role in combining knowledge of effectiveness with patient values and patient circumstances (adapted from Haynes *et al.* [65]).

require reform. EBM publications do not tell clinicians how to integrate patient values and circumstances with the best clinical research. Similarly, most EBM workshops focus on critical appraisal of clinical research and spend little (if any) time telling clinicians how to learn about or integrate patient values and circumstances into their clinical decision-making.

A minimum requirement for integrating patient values and circumstances with the best research evidence would surely involve active empathetic listening of the type conducted by psychological ("talking") therapists. This type of listening is currently not emphasized in most countries. In the UK, for example, general practitioners are recommended to spend no more than 10 minutes [530] with their patients. An empirical study revealed that the average time general practitioners spend with patients is 9.4 minutes (with a standard deviation of 4.7 minutes) [531]. This might be insufficient time to get a clear picture of the individual patient's values and circumstances. Some authors have argued that the limited time general practitioners have with their patients leads to overuse of expensive tests and, ultimately, worse outcomes [532]. EBM in particular has been criticized for failing to emphasize the role of listening to patients in clinical practice [64].

In fact, there is convincing evidence that increasing the time doctors spend with their patients has an independent therapeutic benefit, perhaps by enhancing what is sometimes called the placebo effect.

11.4.2 Expertise is required to enhance the placebo effect

A recent study has quantified the therapeutic benefit of a clinician's contact with patients. Kaptchuk *et al.* [258] compared three groups of patients with IBS. Each group received a different "treatment."

1 *Waiting list*. The participants in this group were observed once at the outset of the study and once at the end (after 6 weeks). Outcome in this group was due to natural history of the disease plus potential Hawthorne effects (effects of knowing that one is taking part in a study).

2 *Limited interaction*. Participants in this group received a placebo acupuncture treatment involving the Streitberger needle (a needle that does not actually penetrate the skin) with limited interaction with a practitioner. The limited patient–practitioner relationship was established on the first visit of less than 5 minutes. The practitioners then explained that this was a scientific study and had been instructed not to converse with patients. The outcome in this group was due to natural history plus potential Hawthorne effects plus limited interaction plus any other effects of placebo acupuncture.

3 *Augmented interaction*. Participants in this group received the same placebo acupuncture treatment as group 2, but had more extensive contact with the practitioners. The initial visit lasted 45 minutes and was structured with respect to both content and style. Content included questions concerning symptoms, how IBS related to relationships and lifestyle, possible non-gastrointestinal symptoms, and how the patient understood his or her condition. The interviewer incorporated at least five primary behaviors, including a warm friendly manner; active listening and empathy (such as saying "I can understand how difficult IBS must be for you"); 20 seconds of thoughtful silence whilst feeling the pulse or pondering the treatment plan; and communication of confidence and positive expectation ("I have had much positive experience treating IBS and look forward to demonstrating that acupuncture is a valuable treatment in this trial"). Specific cognitive and behavioral interventions that might be beneficial for IBS (such as relaxation, cognitive behavioral therapy, or education/counselling) were not allowed. The outcome in this group was due to natural history plus Hawthorne effects plus augmented interaction plus any other effects of placebo acupuncture.

The investigators found a significant increase in all outcomes as the length and "intensity" of the consultation increased ($P < 0.001$). They conclude, "such factors as warmth, empathy, duration of interaction, and the communication of positive expectation might indeed significantly affect

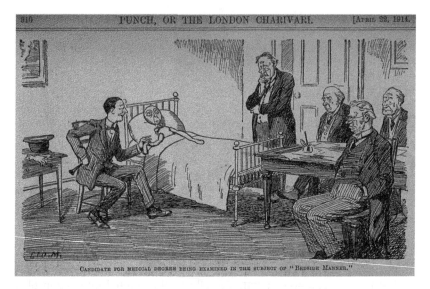

Figure 11.5 Experts as a therapeutic agent (Wellcome image no. 11760).

clinical outcome" and that "nonspecific effects have a considerable clinical impact" [258].

There is some debate about whether the augmented consultation should have been classified as a placebo. Some have suggested that the augmented consultation was in fact a form of cognitive behavior therapy or psychodynamic–interpersonal therapy [323,533]. While I agree with this objection [333], the salient issue here is that, for IBS, and presumably for many other ailments, a caring clinician who empathizes and takes time with their patient can have a positive therapeutic impact on the outcome.

One might also object that many ailments do not seem to be influenced by placebo [168,169]. For example, empathetic and lengthy consultations may not have a huge effect on acute appendicitis or meningitis. Yet even when ailments are unlikely to be placebo responsive, a sympathetic clinician could affect more general – and, arguably, equally important – outcomes such as making a patient feel good. Archie Cochrane recounts the following true story about one of his experiences as the only doctor in a prisoner-of-war camp during the Second World War (Figure 11.5).

> The Germans dumped a young Soviet prisoner in my ward late one night. The ward was full, so I put him in my room as he was moribund

and screaming and I did not want to wake the ward. I examined him.
He had obvious gross bilateral cavitations and severe pleural rub. I
thought the latter was the cause of the pain and screaming. I had no
morphia, just aspirin, which had no effect. I felt desperate. I knew
very little Russian then and there was no one in the ward who did.
I finally instinctively sat down on the bed and took him in my arms,
and the screaming stopped almost at once. He died peacefully in my
arms a few hours later. It was not the pleurisy that caused the screaming but loneliness. It was a wonderful education about the care of
the dying. I was ashamed of my misdiagnosis and kept the story
secret [492].

Many of us no doubt are aware of much less dramatic examples. I once
experienced severe knee pain and inflammation after doing single legged
squats. I visited my doctor who examined me and assured me it was a
sprained ligament that would get better with time. His reassurance certainly alleviated any worry about my knee and even seemed to reduce
the pain. In short, a clinician who consciously empathizes and takes more
time with their patient can have a positive therapeutic impact whether the
outcome in question is placebo responsive or not.

11.4.3 Skills are required to perform any of the skills required in gathering, appraising, and implementing evidence

I have two retired racing greyhounds. A few years ago, one of them
was limping on his rear right leg, and the "normal" veterinary surgeon
took X-rays (under general anesthesia which is far more risky for dogs
than for humans) on several occasions but could neither diagnose nor
treat the problem satisfactorily. I eventually tracked down a greyhound
physiotherapist who, after no more than 30 seconds of examination,
diagnosed the problem (a sprained ligament caused by racing around
the racing track in the same direction) and gave me a treatment (an anti-
inflammatory cream used primarily by racehorses) that made the limp
disappear within hours and never returned. The greyhound physiotherapist had a great deal of expertise with racing greyhounds that the regular
vet simply did not possess.

Likewise, designing and conducting clinical trials, taking blood pressure,
eliciting an accurate case history, examining a patient, and performing surgical operations are skills that, like driving a car or riding a bicycle, require
tacit knowledge [534,535], experience and deliberate practice to master.
Expert tacit knowledge is also required to consider and weigh patient
values and circumstances with the best external evidence and to maximize

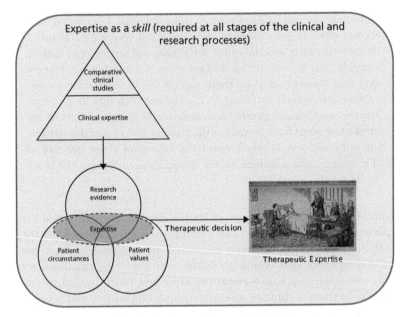

Figure 11.6 Expertise as essential for designing, and conducting clinical research.

the placebo effect. As a skill, expertise pervades all aspects of clinical decision-making and research processes (Figure 11.6).

11.5 Conclusion

...it's about a quarter-century since we discovered that a formula can trounce a physician if you're prepared to do a little work identifying the variables. How many such formulae have been produced by the prodigal colossus of medical research since then? How many systematic efforts have been made to find them? Silence speaks louder than words.

—M. SCRIVEN [508]

EBM advocates are correct to warn against the evidential value of authoritative pronouncements and expert judgment as reliable sources of knowledge *that* therapies are effective either for groups or individuals. A vast body of evidence, backed up by a strong theoretical rationale, indicates that using expert judgment to make predictions about diagnosis, prognosis, or therapeutic benefit results in substandard medical care.

However, expertise is required to play several other, equally important roles, including integrating patient values and circumstances, maximizing the therapeutic benefit of a treatment, and performing various other skills requiring the tacit knowledge of an expert. These other roles for expertise do not belong within a hierarchy of evidence, but rather alongside a hierarchy of evidence. Indeed the characterization of EBM should change from "Evidence-based medicine (EBM) requires the integration of the best research evidence with our clinical expertise and our patient's unique values and circumstances" [34] to:

> EBM requires clinical expertise for producing and interpreting evidence, performing clinical skills, and integrating the best research evidence with patient values and circumstances.

The correct roles for expertise imply that several changes must be made to current medical education and EBM workshops in order to produce the best experts. EBM proponents are correct that more time must be spent learning how to search for and appraise the best evidence. And as it is important to integrate patient values and circumstances with the best evidence, expert clinicians must be allowed to place greater emphasis on listening attentively and empathetically to their patients.

If experts are to maximize placebo effects, then more time needs to be spent with patients. In the past, doctors spent much more time with their patients and often had a remarkable bedside manner. The additional time and empathy no doubt allowed those doctors to learn far more about their patients' circumstances at home and at work than current doctors know. As Kaptchuk's study suggests, this knowledge may have had therapeutic benefits of its own. Unfortunately, that additional knowledge of circumstances and values rarely helped success rates in the past because few effective treatments were available, and many doctors simply did not know how to use those treatments that were available. Now the pendulum may have swung too far the other way. Contemporary doctors have access to an arsenal of powerful treatments yet may lack the time to enhance the placebo effect or to incorporate equally important knowledge about their patients' values and circumstances into clinical decisions.

PART IV
Conclusions

CHAPTER 12

Moving EBM forward

12.1 Summary of findings: the EBM philosophy is acceptable, but . . .

This book has three simple arguments. First, I argued that the EBM requirement that systematic reviews of "best" research evidence should inform clinical decisions is uncontroversial. Strange as it may seem, pre-EBM "methods" for determining whether treatments were effective rarely required formally that clinical decisions be informed by best current evidence. Second, I contended that the EBM view of what counts as best evidence requires some modification. In brief, I argued that the EBM hierarchy, while usually defensible, leads to several paradoxes that can be resolved by replacing the hierarchy with the criterion that all sufficiently high-quality evidence be weighed together in support of a hypothesis that a treatment caused a patient-relevant outcome. Third, the features of being double masked or employing placebo are far less straightforward than many have supposed; once analyzed carefully it is clear that neither plays its intended function reliably. I will now review these conclusions in slightly more detail.

EBM proponents are correct that randomized trials suffer from fewer confounders than observational studies. Yet a categorical ranking of randomized trials over observational studies leads to the paradox of effectiveness, whereby best evidence does not seem to support the effects of our most dramatically effective therapies. The paradox can be resolved by replacing strict hierarchies with a requirement that comparative clinical studies reveal an effect size that outweighs the combined effect of plausible confounders. This requirement would allow observational studies to provide equally strong evidence to randomized trials in some cases, and would

The Philosophy of Evidence-Based Medicine, First Edition. Jeremy Howick.
© 2011 Jeremy Howick. Published 2011 by Blackwell Publishing Ltd.

also be more exacting of certain randomized trials. Rather than display-ing some (statistically significant) benefit, randomized trials would have to reveal a minimum effect size before being accepted as sufficiently strong evidence. LIkewise, observational studies whose effect size outweighs the combined effect of plausible confounders can provide strong evidential support.

While double masking is *often* a methodological virtue because it rules out confounders, unsuccessful masking caused by dramatic effects does not serve any purpose. Meanwhile, treatments labeled as placebo controls often do not perform their function of isolating the characteristic effects of a treatment. I argued that placebos are best characterized as treatments in their own right; viewed as such, it is clear that the assertion that PCTs are methodologically superior to ACTs is difficult to maintain.

EBM proponents are also correct that various often overlooked problems plague mechanistic reasoning. Yet not all mechanistic reasoning was cre-ated equal. High-quality mechanistic reasoning involving inferences from "not incomplete" mechanisms that take into account complexity can and should be allowed to bolster the strength of evidence in favor of claims that treatments are effective. In some cases, high-quality mechanistic reasoning will sometimes be sufficient to support claims that treatments produced clinically relevant benefits, and will be able to bolster evidence from com-parative clinical studies.

Finally, EBM advocates are correct to warn against the evidential value of authoritative pronouncements and expert judgment as reliable sources of knowledge *that* therapies are effective. A vast body of evidence, backed up by a strong theoretical rationale, indicates that using expert judgment when strong evidence exists results in poorer outcomes. At the same time, expertise is required to play several other equally important roles. These include integrating patient values and circumstances with external evi-dence, maximizing the therapeutic benefit of a treatment, and performing various other skills that require the tacit knowledge of an expert. With that in mind, I suggested that the characterization of EBM should change from "Evidence-based medicine (EBM) requires the integration of the best research evidence with our clinical expertise and our patient's unique val-ues and circumstances" [34] to:

> EBM requires clinical expertise for producing and interpreting evi-dence, performing clinical skills, and integrating the best research evi-dence with patient values and circumstances.

The EBM philosophy of evidence, even with my suggested modifications, has implications for how treatments are appraised, as well as how medicine is taught and practiced. Immediately before the EBM movement became popular, a common method for determining whether treatments had their putative effects were consensus meetings where experts would gather around a table and decide whether a new agent was effective [103,104–110]. Now EBM requires experts to systematically and transparently appraise the evidence upon which their recommendations are based. Likewise, medical education is centered around the primal importance of mechanistic knowledge and expertise. Medical training generally involves 2–3 years of preclinical studies, where students primarily learn pathology and physiology, followed by 2–3 years where they follow more senior "experts" in what could be described as an apprenticeship method. EBM proponents recommend modifying the curriculum to emphasize the importance of searching for, and appraising, clinical evidence.

12.2 Two new frontiers for EBM

12.2.1 The next step in critical appraisal: the hidden biases caused by conflict of interest

While the EBM movement has made great strides in improving the quality of comparative clinical studies [234,261], a new class of biases have become increasingly apparent. The new problem (it is not really new, but merely has become more evident recently) is that industry-sponsored trials are more likely to show a beneficial effect than non-industry funded trials [261,536–540). This is strange since both industry and publicly sponsored trials seem to be of the same quality – both employ concealed random allocation and (where appropriate and feasible) double masking, and often have the same endpoints. This bias can have paradoxical consequences. For example, Heres *et al.* [541] examined randomized trials that compared different antipsychotic medications. They found that olanzapine beat risperidone, risperidone beat quetiapine, and quetiapine beat olanzapine! The relative success of the drugs was directly related to who sponsored the trial. For example, if the manufacturers of risperidone sponsored the trial, then risperidone was more likely to appear more effective than the others. There are political [84], sociological [542], and methodological solutions to these new biases. I will briefly discuss the three potential methodological solutions since these are more clearly within the EBM remit to rectify.

The first (mostly) methodological reason why industry-sponsored studies (or, presumably, any study sponsored by a person or group with a strong personal or financial interest in a particular outcome) might be more likely to reveal a benefit of their drug is publication bias. It is usually against a pharmaceutical company's interest to publish trials where their drugs did not demonstrate an effect. It is therefore hardly surprising that positive results are more likely to be published than negative results [543]. To cite one example, Turner *et al.* [544] examined all the antidepressant trials registered by the FDA. They identified 74 studies, 38 (51%) with positive results and 36 with negative or questionable results. Of the trials with positive results, all but one were published, whereas of the 36 trials with negative results, 22 were unpublished. To overcome this problem many advocate mandatory registration of clinical studies [545]. If trials must be registered, it is more difficult (but not impossible) to suppress trials with negative results.

The problem with publication bias is exacerbated by duplicate publications. Sometimes the same study will be published in more than one journal with different authors. Tramer *et al.* [546] found that 17% of studies and 38% of patient data were duplicated, and (unsurprisingly) the likelihood of being duplicated was increased if the trial results were positive. In one example, nine trials of ondansetron (an antiemetic) were published in 14 reports with no clear cross-referencing. Failure to spot the duplicate publication would lead to a 23% overestimation of ondansetron's positive effects in a systematic review [546]. The methodological solution to duplicate publications might simply be to require that it be cross-referenced.

The second methodological reason industry-sponsored trials are more likely to demonstrate a benefit is bias that enters during the data-analysis phase of a study. Many prominent researchers have acknowledged in confidential conversations that they hire two or three statisticians to analyze data. A data analyst, knowing what result the lead investigator prefers, might have a personal or professional interest in making the lead investigator's desired outcome more likely. One obvious way a statistician can influence the results is to purposefully, or more charitably erroneously, make a calculation error to make a treatment appear more effective than a control when in fact it is not. In fact, there is strong evidence that data analysts can influence the report of a study. In an interesting study Peter Gøtzsche analyzed trial reports of 196 trials comparing new NSAIDs with established NSAIDs. He found that the new drugs were five times more likely to appear more effective than the established drugs. This was surprising based on historical evidence that NSAIDs are, on average, equally effective [547,548]. Where possible, Gøtzsche reanalyzed the data and found that the apparent benefits of the new drugs were errors, and in all cases the erroneous reporting of results favored the new drugs. Gøtzsche also found that calculations of side-effects were biased [548]. This was achieved by selectively including or excluding patients who had withdrawn due to side-effects in the analysis. An obvious solution to the problem of biased data analysis is to mask the data analysts [549]. If data analysts did not know which was the experimental therapy, they would not be able to predictably make systematic errors or omissions that favored the apparent benefit of the experimental drug.

However, masking the data analysts would not suffice. In some cases trials suggest no benefit of a new drug, but the trial report is written as if the drug were beneficial. In Turner *et al.*'s review of antidepressant trials cited above, 11 of the 36 negative trials were presented in a way that conveyed a positive outcome. This means that a naive review of the published antidepressant trials would suggest that 94% indicated a positive result whereas in fact only about half (51%) suggested that the drugs had a beneficial effect. The difference here is between virtual unanimity (94%) and a coin toss (51%). Other studies have replicated this finding [536]. In one interesting study, Stelfox *et al.* [550] examined the relationship between likelihood to support the effects of calcium channel antagonists and their financial relationships with the pharmaceutical industry. They found that 96% of supportive authors had a financial relationship with the manufacturer, compared with 60% of neutral authors and 37% of critical authors.

To recap, a "new" level of critical appraisal is required to address the biases that enter during the data analysis, publication, and manuscript authoring phases. This can be at least partially resolved by insisting on trial registration and masking the data analysts and manuscript authors.

12.2.2 Applying EBM to the big picture

In Chapters 5, 10, and 11 I cited examples where randomized trials revealed the uselessness or harm caused by many treatments that had been introduced by observational studies (HRT) or mechanistic reasoning (antiarrhythmic drugs). Provided that we believe the results of the randomized trials are more reliable (and I argued that we should), it seems that EBM saves lives. But when it comes to improving health outcomes, medical treatment is not the only game in town. Some have argued that improved economic conditions rather than medical treatments caused at least *some* of the reduction in infant mortality and increase in life expectancy in the last century [96]. More recently, Wilkinson and Marmot [551] have been catalysts for a research program that has provided persuasive evidence that social factors rather than medical treatment are the cause of good health. Given that healthcare resources are scarce, it is useful to know which "intervention" (medical treatment, improved economic conditions, increased equality, or some combination of these) has the biggest effect. In fact, we saw in the discussion of non-inferiority trials in Chapter 8 that it is possible to exploit the EBM methodology to increase healthcare spending without improving patient outcomes.

This is not a criticism of EBM, but rather a question about whether medical treatments are the most efficient way to improve health outcomes. At the same time, given that there are alternatives, it would be useful for EBM proponents to develop robust methodologies for evaluating the relative effects of the different options available for improving overall health.

References

1 Ashcroft R, ter Meulen R. Ethics, philosophy, and evidence based medicine. *Journal of Medical Ethics* 2004;30:119.

2 Hill AB, Hill ID. *Bradford Hill's Principles of Medical Statistics*, 12th edn. London: Edward Arnold, 1991.

3 Popper KR. *The Logic of Scientific Discovery*. London: Hutchinson, 1959. Revised edition 1968.

4 Djulbegovic B, Guyatt GH, Ashcroft RE. Epistemologic inquiries in evidence-based medicine. *Cancer Control* 2009;16:158–68.

5 Sehon SR, Stanley DE. A philosophical analysis of the evidence-medicine debate. *BMC Health Services Research* 2003;3:14–24.

6 Celsus AC. *A Translation of the Eight Books of Aul. Corn. Celsus on Medicine*. Translated by GF Collier. London: Simpkin and Marshall, 1831.

7 Avicenna. *Al Qānūn. The Canon*. Chicago: Great Books of the Islamic World, 1999.

8 Louis PCA. Researches on the effects of blood letting in some inflammatory diseases, and on the influence of tartarized antimony and vesication in pneumonitis. Translated by CG Putnam, with preface and appendix by J Jackson. Boston: Hillard, Gray, 1836.

9 Bernard C. *An Introduction to the Study of Experimental Medicine*. New York: Dover Publications, 1957.

10 Eddy DM. Practice policies: where do they come from? *Journal of the American Medical Association* 1990;263:1265, 1269, 1272 passim.

11 Guyatt G. Evidence-based medicine. *Americal College of Physicians Journal Club* 1991;114:A16.

12 Evidence Based Medicine Working Group. Evidence-based medicine. A new approach to teaching the practice of medicine. *Journal of the American Medical Association* 1992;268:2420–5.

13 Moher D, Schulz KF, Altman D. The CONSORT statement: revised recommendations for improving the quality of reports of parallel-group randomized trials. *Journal of the American Medical Association* 2001;285:1987–91.

14 Hitt J. The Year in Ideas: A to Z; Evidence-Based Medicine. *The New York Times* December 9, 2001, section 68.

15 The Campbell Collaboration. Available at www.campbellcollaboration.org/ [accessed September 30, 2009]

16 O'Connor TS. The search for truth: the case for evidence based chaplaincy. *Journal of Health Care Chaplaincy* 2002;13:185–94.

17 *The Oxford English Dictionary*, 2nd edn. Oxford: Oxford University Press, 1989.

18 Canadian Task Force on the Periodic Health Examination. The periodic health examination. *Canadian Medical Association Journal* 1979;121:1193–254.

19 Guyatt GH, Oxman AD, Vist GE *et al.* GRADE: an emerging consensus on rating quality of evidence and strength of recommendations. *British Medical Journal* 2008;336:924–6.

20 Harbour RT (ed.) *SIGN 50: A Guideline Developer's Handbook.* Edinburgh: NHS Quality Improvement Scotland, 2008.

21 Phillips B, Ball C, Sackett D *et al. Oxford Centre for Evidence-based Medicine Levels of Evidence.* Oxford: CEBM, 2001. Available from www.cebm.net/?o=1021

22 Sackett DL. Rules of evidence and clinical recommendations on the use of antithrombotic agents. *Chest* 1986;89(2 Suppl.):2S–3S.

23 Sackett DL. Rules of evidence and clinical recommendations on the use of antithrombotic agents. *Chest* 1989;95(2 Suppl.):2S–4S.

24 Evans I, Thornton H, Chalmers I. *Testing Treatments: Better Research for Better Healthcare.* London: British Library, 2006.

25 Healy D. *Let Them Eat Prozac.* New York: New York University Press, 2004.

26 Healy D. Did regulators fail over selective serotonin reuptake inhibitors? *British Medical Journal* 2006;333:92–5.

27 Kirsch I, Sapirstein G. Listening to Prozac but hearing placebo: a meta-analysis of antidepressant medication. *Prevention and Treatment.* 1998.

28 Kirsch I, Moore T. The emperor's new drugs: an analysis of antidepressant medication data submitted to the U.S. Food and Drug Administration. *Prevention and Treatment.* 2002.

29 Moncrieff J, Kirsch I. Efficacy of antidepressants in adults. *British Medical Journal* 2005;331:155–7.

30 Smith GC, Pell JP. Parachute use to prevent death and major trauma related to gravitational challenge: systematic review of randomised controlled trials. *British Medical Journal* 2003;327:1459–61.

31 Glasziou P, Chalmers I, Rawlins M, McCulloch P. When are randomised trials unnecessary? Picking signal from noise. *British Medical Journal* 2007;334:349–51.

32 Sackett DL, Richardson WS, Rosenberg W, Haynes B. *Evidence-based Medicine: How to Practice and Teach EBM.* London: Churchill Livingstone, 1997.

33 Sackett DL. *Evidence-based Medicine: How to Practice and Teach EBM,* 2nd edn. Edinburgh: Churchill Livingstone, 2000.

34 Straus SE, Richardson WS, Glasziou P, Haynes RB. *Evidence-based Medicine: How to Practice and Teach EBM,* 3rd edn. London: Elsevier, Churchill Livingstone, 2005.

35 Barton S. Which clinical studies provide the best evidence? The best RCT still trumps the best observational study. *British Medical Journal* 2000;321:255–6.

36 Benson K, Hartz AJ. A comparison of observational studies and randomized, controlled trials. *New England Journal of Medicine* 2000;342:1878–86.

37 Cartwright N. Are RCTs the gold standard? *Biosocieties* 2007; 2:11–20.

38 Concato J, Shah N, Horwitz RI. Randomized, controlled trials, observational studies, and the hierarchy of research designs. *New England Journal of Medicine* 2000;342:1887–92.

39 Concato J. Observational versus experimental studies: what's the evidence for a hierarchy? *NeuroRx* 2004;1:341–7.

40 Grossman J, MacKenzie F. The randomized controlled trial: gold standard, or merely standard? *Perspectives in Biology and Medicine* 2005;48:516–34.

41 La Caze A. Evidence-based medicine must be. *Journal of Medicine and Philosophy* 2009;34:509–27.

42 Morrison K. Randomised controlled trials for evidence-based education: some problems in judging "what works". *Evaluation and Research in Education* 2001;15:69–83.

43 Penston J. *Fact and Fiction in Medical Research: The Large-Scale Randomised Trial.* London: The London Press, 2003.

44 Pocock SJ, Elbourne DR. Randomized trials or observational tribulations? *New England Journal of Medicine* 2000;342:1907–9.

45 Sacks H, Chalmers TC, Smith H Jr. Randomized versus historical controls for clinical trials. *American Journal of Medicine* 1982;72:233–40.

46 Worrall J. *What* evidence in evidence-based medicine? *Philosophy of Science* 2002;69(Suppl.):S316–S330.

47 Worrall J. Evidence in medicine. *Compass* 2007;2:981–1022.

48 Worrall J. Why there's no cause to randomize. *British Journal for the Philosophy of Science* 2007;58:451–88.

49 Howson C, Urbach P. *Scientific Reasoning: the Bayesian Approach*, 2nd edn. Illinois: Open Court, 1993.

50 Lindley DV. The role of randomization in inference. *Proceedings of the Biennial Meeting of the Philosophy of Science Association* 1982;2:431–46.

51 Bluhm R. From hierarchy to network: a richer view of evidence for evidence-based medicine. *Perspectives in Biology and Medicine* 2005;48: 535–47.

52 Cartwright N, Goldfinch A, Howick J (eds) *Evidence-based Policy: Where is Our Theory of Evidence?* Milan: Graduate Conference of the Graduate School for Social Sciences, 2007.

53 Cartwright N. *Causal Powers: What Are They? Why Do We Need Them? What Can Be Done With Them and What Cannot?* London: Centre for the Philosophy of Natural and Social Science, 2007.

54 Cartwright N. Presidential address. American Philosophical Association Pacific Division, Vancouver, April 10, 2009.

55 Gillies D. In defense of the Popper–Miller argument. *Philosophy of Science* 1986;53(111).

56 La Caze A. The role of basic science in evidence based medicine. *Biology and Philosophy* 2009;26(1):81–98.

57 Maclure M. Mechanistic versus empirical explanations and evidence-based medicine. *Acta Oncologica* 1998;37:11–13.

58 Tobin MJ. Counterpoint: evidence-based medicine lacks a sound scientific base. *Chest* 2008;133:1071–4; discussion 4–7.

59 Tonelli MR. The philosophical limits of evidence-based medicine. *Academic Medicine* 1998;73:1234–40.

60 Tonelli MR. The limits of evidence-based medicine. *Respiratory Care* 2001;46:1435–40; discussion 40–1.

61 Tonelli MR. Integrating evidence into clinical practice: an alternative to evidence-based approaches. *Journal of Evaluation in Clinical Practice* 2006;12:248–56.

62 Mant D. Can randomised trials inform clinical decisions about individual patients? *Lancet* 1999;353:743–6.

63 Upshur RE, Colak E. Argumentation and evidence. *Theoretical Medicine and Bioethics* 2003;24:283–99.

64 Upshur R. Looking for rules in a world of exceptions: reflections on evidence-based practice. *Perspectives in Biology and Medicine* 2005;48:477–89.

65 Haynes RB, Devereaux PJ, Guyatt GH. Clinical expertise in the era of evidence-based medicine and patient choice. *Americal College of Physicians Journal Club* 2002;136:A11–A14.

66 Englehardt HTJ, Spicker SF, Towers B (eds) *Clinical Judgment: A Critical Appraisal*. Dordrecht: D. Reidel Publishing Company, 1977.

67 Timmermans S. From autonomy to accountability: the role of clinical practice guidelines in professional power. *Perspectives in Biology and Medicine* 2005;48:490–501.

68 Borgerson K. Evidence-based alternative medicine? *Perspectives in Biology and Medicine* 2005;48:502–15.

69 Vandenbroucke JP. Alternative treatments in reproductive medicine. The vexing problem of "seemingly impeccable trials". *Human Reproduction* 2002;17:2228–9.

70 Vandenbroucke JP, de Craen AJ. Alternative medicine: a "mirror image" for scientific reasoning in conventional medicine. *Annals of Internal Medicine* 2001;135:507–13.

71 Goodman KW. *Ethics and Evidence-based Medicine: Fallibility and Responsibility in Clinical Science*. Cambridge: Cambridge University Press, 2003.

72 Goodman KW. Ethics, evidence, and public policy. *Perspectives in Biology and Medicine* 2005;48:548–56.

73 Goldenberg MJ. Evidence-based ethics? On evidence-based practice and the "empirical turn" from normative bioethics. *BMC Medical Ethics* 2005;6:E11.

74 Howick J. Questioning the methodologic superiority of "placebo" over "active" controlled trials. *American Journal of Bioethics* 2009;9:34–48.

75 McGuire WL. Beyond EBM: new directions for evidence-based public health. *Perspectives in Biology and Medicine* 2005;48:557–69.

76 Dopson S. Evidence-based medicine and the implementation gap. *Health: An Interdisciplinary Journal for the Social Study of Health, Illness and Medicine* 2003;7:311–30.

77 Timmermans S, Mauck A. The promises and pitfalls of evidence-based medicine. *Health Affairs (Millwood)* 2005;24:18–28.

78 Daly J. *Evidence-based Medicine and the Search for a Science of Clinical Care*. Berkeley: University of California Press, 2005.

79 Pope C. Resisting the evidence: the study of evidence-based medicine as a contemporary social movement. *Health: An Interdisciplinary Journal for the Social Study of Health, Illness and Medicine* 2003;7:267–82.

80 Goldenberg MJ. On evidence and evidence-based medicine: lessons from the philosophy of science. *Social Science and Medicine* 2006;62:2621–32.

81 Holmes D, Murray S, Perron A, Rail G. Deconstructing the evidence-based discourse in health sciences: truth, power and fascism. *International Journal of Evidence-Based Healthcare* 2006;4:180–6.

82 Ashcroft RE. Current epistemological problems in evidence based medicine. *Journal of Medical Ethics* 2004;30:131–5.

83 Freedman B. Equipoise and the ethics of clinical research. *New England Journal of Medicine* 1987;317:141–5.

84 Brown JR. Politics, method, and medical research. *Philosophy of Science* 2008;75:756–66.

85 Asher R. *Talking Sense*. London: Pitman Medical, 1972.

86 Matthews R. Almroth Wright, vaccine therapy, and British biometrics: disciplinary expertise versus statistical objectivity. *Clio Medica* 2002;67:125–47.

87 Tröhler U. *To Improve the Evidence of Medicine: The 18th Century British Origins of a Critical Approach*. Royal College of Physicians of Edinburgh, 2001.

88 Gillies D. Debates on Bayesianism and the theory of Bayesian networks. *Theoria* 1998;64:1–22.

89 Gillies D. Hempelian and Kuhnian approaches in the philosophy of medicine: the Semmelweis case. *Studies in the History and Philosophy of Biological and Biomedical Sciences* 2005;36:159–81.

90 Dawes M, Summerskill W, Glasziou P *et al*. Sicily statement on evidence-based practice. *BMC Medical Education* 2005;5:1.

91 Guyatt G, Cook D, Haynes B. Evidence based medicine has come a long way. *British Medical Journal* 2004;329:990–1.

92 Sackett DL, Rosenberg WM, Gray JA, Haynes RB, Richardson WS. Evidence based medicine: what it is and what it isn't. *British Medical Journal* 1996;312:71–2.

93 Straus SE. What's the E for EBM? *British Medical Journal* 2004;328:535–6.

94 LeFanu J. *The Rise and Fall of Modern Medicine*. London: Abacus, 2000.

95 Horder. Whither medicine? *British Medical Journal* 1949;1(4604):557–60.

96 McKeown T. *The Role of Medicine: Dream, Mirage or Nemesis?* London: Nuffield Provincial Hospitals Trust, 1976.

97 Illich I. *Limits to Medicine. Medical Nemesis: the Expropriation of Health*. Harmondsworth: Penguin, 1977.

98 Chalmers I. Why we need to know whether prophylactic antibiotics can reduce measles-related morbidity. *Pediatrics* 2002;109:312–15.

99 Sackett D. A 1955 clinical trial report that changed my career. James Lind Library, 2008 (http://www.jameslindlibrary.org/).

100 Sackett DL. Clinical epidemiology. *American Journal of Epidemiology* 1969;89:125–8.

101 Sackett DL, Haynes B, Tugwell P (eds) *Clinical Epidemiology: A Basic Science for Clinical Medicine*, 2nd edn. Boston: Little, Brown, 1985.

102 Guyatt G. (personal communication).

103 Goodman C, Baratz SR (eds) *Improving Consensus Development for Health Technology Assessment: An International Perspective*. Washington, DC: National Academy Press, 1990.

104 Battista RN. Profile of a Consensus Development Program in Canada: the Canadian Task Force on the Periodic Health Examination. In: Goodman C, Baratz SR (eds) *Improving Consensus Development for Health Technology Assessment: An International Perspective.* Washington, DC: National Academy Press, 1990, pp. 87–92.

105 Jørgensen T. Profile of a Consensus Development Program in Denmark: the Danish Medical Reseasrch Council and the Danish Hospital Institute. In: Goodman C, Baratz SR (eds) *Improving Consensus Development for Health Technology Assessment: An International Perspective.* Washington, DC: National Academy Press, 1990, pp. 96–101.

106 Kauppila A-L. Profile of a Consensus Development Program in Finland: the Medical Research Council of the Academy of Finland. In: Goodman C, Baratz SR (eds) *Improving Consensus Development for Health Technology Assessment: An International Perspective.* Washington, DC: National Academy Press, 1990, pp. 102–9.

107 Kazinga NS, Casparie AF, Everdingen JJE. Profile of a Consensus Development Program in Finland: National Organization for Quality Assurance in Hospitals. In: Goodman C, Baratz SR (eds) *Improving Consensus Development for Health Technology Assessment: An International Perspective.* Washington, DC: National Academy Press, 1990, pp. 110–17.

108 Backe B. Profile of a Consensus Development Program in Norway: the Norwegian Institute for Hospital Research and the National Research Council. In: Goodman C, Baratz SR (eds) *Improving Consensus Development for Health Technology Assessment: An International Perspective.* Washington, DC: National Academy Press, 1990, pp. 118–24.

109 Håkansoon S, Eckerlund I. Profile of a Consensus Development Program in Sweden: the Swedish Medical Research Council and the Swedish Planning and Rationalization Institute for the Health and Social Services. In: Goodman C, Baratz SR (eds) *Improving Consensus Development for Health Technology Assessment: An International Perspective.* Washington, DC: National Academy Press, 1990, pp. 125–30.

110 Spilby J. Profile of a Consensus Development Program in the United Kingdom: The King's Fund Forum. In: Goodman C, Baratz SR (eds) *Improving Consensus Development for Health Technology Assessment: An International Perspective.* Washington, DC: National Academy Press, 1990, pp. 131–6.

111 Antman EM, Lau J, Kupelnick B, Mosteller F, Chalmers TC. A comparison of results of meta-analyses of randomized control trials and recommendations of clinical experts. Treatments for myocardial infarction. *Journal of the American Medical Association* 1992;268:240–8.

112 The Cardiac Arrhythmia Suppression Trial (CAST) Investigators. Preliminary report: effect of encainide and flecainide on mortality in a randomized trial of arrhythmia suppression after myocardial infarction. *New England Journal of Medicine* 1989;321:406–12.

113 The Cardiac Arrhythmia Suppression Trial II Investigators. Effect of the antiarrhythmic agent moricizine on survival after myocardial infarction. *New England Journal of Medicine* 1992;327:227–33.

114 Anon. How to read clinical journals. V: To distinguish useful from useless or even harmful therapy. *Canadian Medical Association Journal* 1981;124: 1156–62.

115 Carnap R. On the application of inductive logic. *International Phenomenological Society* 1947;8:133–48.

116 Crowley PA. Corticosteroids in pregnancy: the benefits outweight the costs. *Journal of Obstetrics and Gynaecology* 1981;1:147–50.

117 Liggins GC, Howie RN. A controlled trial of antepartum glucocorticoid treatment for prevention of the respiratory distress syndrome in premature infants. *Pediatrics* 1972;50:515–25.

118 Block MF, Kling OR, Crosby WM. Antenatal glucocorticoid therapy for the prevention of respiratory distress syndrome in the premature infant. *Obstetrics and Gynecology* 1977;50:186–90.

119 Papageorgiou AN, Desgranges MF, Masson M, Colle E, Shatz R, Gelfand MM. The antenatal use of betamethasone in the prevention of respiratory distress syndrome: a controlled double-blind study. *Pediatrics* 1979;63:73–9.

120 Taeusch HW Jr, Frigoletto F, Kitzmiller J *et al.* Risk of respiratory distress syndrome after prenatal dexamethasone treatment. *Pediatrics* 1979;63:64–72.

121 Crowley PA. Promoting pulmonary maturity. In: Chalmers I, Enkin M, Keirse MJNC (eds) *Effective Care in Pregnancy and Childbirth.* Oxford: Oxford University Press, 1989, pp. 746–64.

122 Prenatal corticosteroids for reducing morbidity and mortality after preterm birth. Witness Seminar held by the Wellcome Trust Centre for the History of Medicine, 2004.

123 Canadian Task Force on the Periodic Health Examination. The periodic health examination. *Canadian Medical Association Journal* 1979;121:1193–254.

124 Lacchetti C, Ioannidis JP, Guyatt G. Surprising results of randomized, controlled trials. In: Guyatt G, Rennie D (eds) *The Users' Guides to the Medical Literature: A Manual for Evidence-Based Clinical Practice.* Chicago, IL: AMA Publications, 2002.

125 Chalmers I. The lethal consequences of failing to make full use of all relevant evidence about the effects of medical treatments: the importance of systematic reviews. In: Rothwell PM (ed.) *Treating Individuals: From Randomised Trials to Personalized Medicine.* London: The Lancet, 2007.

126 US Preventive Services Task Force. Guide to clinical preventive services. AHRQ Publication No. 10-05145, August 2010. Agency for Healthcare Research and Quality, Rockville, MD. http://www.ahrq.gov/clinic/pocketgd1011/ [accessed December 21, 2010].

127 Boorse C. Health as a theoretical concept. *Philosophy of Science* 1977;44: 542–73.

128 Boyd KM. Disease, illness, sickness, health, healing and wholeness: exploring some elusive concepts. *Medical Humanities* 2000;26.9–17.

129 Collins H, Pinch T. *Dr Golem: How to Think about Medicine.* London: University of Chicago Press, 2005.

130 Cooper R. Disease. *Studies in the History and Philosophy of Science* 2002;33:263–82.

131 Hofmann B. On the triad disease, illness and sickness. *Journal of Medicine and Philosophy* 2002;27:651–73.

132 Nesse RM. On the difficulty of defining disease: a Darwinian perspective. *Medicine, Health Care and Philosophy* 2001;4:37–46.

133 Wikman A, Marklund S, Alexanderson K. Illness, disease, and sickness absence: an empirical test of differences between concepts of ill health. *Journal of Epidemiology and Community Health* 2005;59:450–4.

134 Ebell MH, Barry HC, Slawson DC, Shaughnessy AF. Finding POEMs in the medical literature. *Journal of Family Practice* 1999;48:350–5.

135 Guyatt G, Montori V, Devereaux PJ, Schunemann H, Bhandari M. Patients at the center: in our practice, and in our use of language. *Americal College of Physicians Journal Club* 2004;140:A11–A12.

136 Vickrey BG. Getting oriented to patient-oriented outcomes. *Neurology* 1999;53:662–3.

137 Ashcroft R. What is clinical effectiveness? *Studies in the History and Philosophy of Biological and Biomedical Sciences* 2002;33:219–33.

138 Bland CS. The Halsted mastectomy: present illness and past history. *Western Journal of Medicine* 1981;134:549–55.

139 Wedgwood KR, Benson EA. Non-tumour morbidity and mortality after modified radical mastectomy. *Annals of the Royal College of Surgeons of England* 1992;74:314–17.

140 Worrall J. Do we need some large, simple randomized trials in medicine? *EPSA Philosophical Issues in the Sciences* 2009, 289–301, 2010.

141 The Long-Term Intervention with Pravastatin in Ischaemic Disease (LIPID) Study Group. Prevention of cardiovascular events and death with pravastatin in patients with coronary heart disease and a broad range of initial cholesterol levels. *New England Journal of Medicine* 1998;339:1349–57.

142 Plehn JF, Davis BR, Sacks FM *et al.* Reduction of stroke incidence after myocardial infarction with pravastatin: the Cholesterol and Recurrent Events (CARE) study. *Circulation* 1999;99:216–23.

143 Gruppo Italiano per lo Studio della Sopravvivenza nell'infarto Miocardico. GISSI-3: effects of lisinopril and transdermal glyceryl trinitrate singly and together on 6-week mortality and ventricular function after acute myocardial infarction. *Lancet* 1994;343:1115–22.

144 Bylund DB, Reed AL. Childhood and adolescent depression: why do children and adults respond differently to antidepressant drugs? *Neurochemistry International* 2007;51:246–53.

145 Deupree JD, Reed AL, Bylund DB. Differential effects of the tricyclic antidepressant desipramine on the density of adrenergic receptors in juvenile and adult rats. *Journal of Pharmacology and Experimental Therapeutics* 2007;321: 770–6.

146 Zimmerman M, Posternak MA, Chelminski I. Symptom severity and exclusion from antidepressant efficacy trials. *Journal of Clinical Psychopharmacology* 2002;22:610–14.

147 Zimmerman M, Mattia JI, Posternak MA. Are subjects in pharmacological treatment trials of depression representative of patients in routine clinical practice? *American Journal of Psychiatry* 2002;159:469–73.

148 Zetin M, Hoepner CT. Relevance of exclusion criteria in antidepressant clinical trials: a replication study. *Journal of Clinical Psychopharmacology* 2007;27: 295–301.

149 Travers J, Marsh S, Williams M *et al*. External validity of randomised controlled trials in asthma: to whom do the results of the trials apply? *Thorax* 2007;62:219–23.

150 Rothwell PM. External validity of randomised controlled trials: "to whom do the results of this trial apply?" *Lancet* 2005;365:82–93.

151 Rothwell PM. Treating individuals 2. Subgroup analysis in randomised controlled trials: importance, indications, and interpretation. *Lancet* 2005;365:176–86.

152 Rothwell PM, Mehta Z, Howard SC, Gutnikov SA, Warlow CP. Treating individuals 3. From subgroups to individuals: general principles and the example of carotid endarterectomy. *Lancet* 2005;365:256–65.

153 Blumenthal JA, Sherwood A, Babyak MA *et al*. Effects of exercise and stress management training on markers of cardiovascular risk in patients with ischemic heart disease: a randomized controlled trial. *Journal of the American Medical Association* 2005;293:1626–34.

154 de Feyter PJ, Serruys PW. Acute haemodynamic effects of the beta 1-adrenoceptor partial agonist xamoterol at rest and during supine exercise in patients with left ventricular dysfunction due to ischaemic heart disease: a double-blind randomized trial. *European Heart Journal* 1990;11(Suppl. A):48–9.

155 Froelicher V, Jensen D, Genter F *et al*. A randomized trial of exercise training in patients with coronary heart disease. *Journal of the American Medical Association* 1984;252:1291–7.

156 Taylor RS, Brown A, Ebrahim S *et al*. Exercise-based rehabilitation for patients with coronary heart disease: systematic review and meta-analysis of randomized controlled trials. *American Journal of Medicine* 2004;116:682–92.

157 Berg A, Konig D, Deibert P, Grathwohl D, Baumstark MW, Franz IW. Effect of an oat bran enriched diet on the atherogenic lipid profile in patients with an increased coronary heart disease risk. A controlled randomized lifestyle intervention study. *Annals of Nutrition and Metabolism* 2003;47:306–11.

158 Iglehart JK. Prioritizing comparative-effectiveness research: IOM recommendations. *New England Journal of Medicine* 2009;361:325–8.

159 Sox HC, Greenfield S. Comparative effectiveness research: a report from the Institute of Medicine. *Annals of Internal Medicine* 2009;151:203–5.

160 Howick J. Oxford Centre for Evidence-Based Medicine Levels of Evidence. Available at www.cebm.net/index.aspx?o=5653 [accessed June 18, 2010]

161 Conan Doyle, Sir Arthur. *The Sign of Four*. Salt Lake City: Project Gutenberg, 2000 [accessed December 21, 2010].

162 Warrell DA, Looareesuwan S, Warrell MJ *et al*. Dexamethasone proves deleterious in cerebral malaria. A double-blind trial in 100 comatose patients. *New England Journal of Medicine* 1982;306:313–19.

163 Prendiville WJ, Harding JE, Elbourne DR, Stirrat GM. The Bristol third stage trial: active versus physiological management of third stage of labour. *British Medical Journal* 1988;297:1295–300.

164 Elbourne D, Harding JE. Hair colour and blood loss [letter]. *Midwives Chronicle and Nursing Notes* 1988;(November):363.

165 Dretske FI. Epistemic operators. *Journal of Philosophy* 1970;67:1007–23.

166 Dretske FI. The pragmatic dimension of knowledge. *Philosophical Studies* 1981;40:363–78.

167 Lewis D. Elusive knowledge. *Australasian Journal of Philosophy* 1996;74: 549–67.

168 Hrobjartsson A, Gøtzsche PC. Is the placebo powerless? An analysis of clinical trials comparing placebo with no treatment. *New England Journal of Medicine* 2001;344:1594–602.

169 Hrobjartsson A, Gøtzsche PC. Is the placebo powerless? Update of a systematic review with 52 new randomized trials comparing placebo with no treatment. *Journal of Internal Medicine* 2004;256:91–100.

170 Mill JS. *A System of Logic, Ratiocinative And Inductive: Being a Connected View of the Principles of Evidence and the Methods of Scientific Investigation*. Toronto: University of Toronto Press, 1973 (1843).

171 Popper KR. *Conjectures and Refutations: The Growth of Scientific Knowledge*. London: Routledge and Kegan Paul, 1969.

172 Hempel CG. *Philosophy of Natural Science*. Englewood Cliffs, NJ: Prentice-Hall, 1966.

173 Howson C. *Induction and the Justification of Belief: Hume's Problem*. Oxford: Clarendon Press, 2000.

174 Bland M. *An Introduction to Medical Statistics*, 3rd edn. Oxford: Oxford University Press, 2000.

175 Djulbegovic B, Kumar A, Soares HP *et al*. Treatment success in cancer: new cancer treatment successes identified in phase 3 randomized controlled trials conducted by the National Cancer Institute-sponsored cooperative oncology groups, 1955 to 2006. *Archives of Internal Medicine* 2008;168: 632–42.

176 Borgerson K. Valuing evidence: bias and the evidence hierarchy of evidence-based medicine. *Perspectives in Biology and Medicine* 2009;52:218–33.

177 Worrall J. Evidence: philosophy of science meets medicine. *Journal of Evaluation in Clinical Practice* 2010;16:35.

178 Howick J, Glasziou P, Aronson JK. The evolution of evidence hierarchies: what can Bradford Hill's "guidelines for causation" contribute? *Journal of the Royal Society of Medicine* 2009;102:186–94.

179 Masur H, Michelis MA, Greene JB *et al*. An outbreak of community-acquired *Pneumocystis carinii* pneumonia: initial manifestation of cellular immune dysfunction. *New England Journal of Medicine* 1981;305:1431–8.

180 Petitti DB, Perlman JA, Sidney S. Noncontraceptive estrogens and mortality: long-term follow-up of women in the Walnut Creek Study. *Obstetrics and Gynecology* 1987;70:289–93.

181 Stampfer MJ, Colditz GA. Estrogen replacement therapy and coronary heart disease: a quantitative assessment of the epidemiologic evidence. *Preventive Medicine* 1991;20:47–63.

182 Coronary Drug Project. Influence of adherence to treatment and response of cholesterol on mortality in the coronary drug project. *New England Journal of Medicine* 1980;303:1038–41.

183 Simpson SH, Eurich DT, Majumdar SR *et al.* A meta-analysis of the association between adherence to drug therapy and mortality. *British Medical Journal* 2006;333:15.

184 Jadad A. *Randomized Controlled Trials.* London: BMJ Books, 1998.

185 Schulz KF. Subverting randomization in controlled trials. *Journal of the American Medical Association* 1995;274:1456–8.

186 Anon. Streptomycin treatment of pulmonary tuberculosis. *British Medical Journal* 1948;2(4582):769–82.

187 Cocco G. Erectile dysfunction after therapy with metoprolol: the Hawthorne effect. *Cardiology* 2009;112:174–7.

188 McCarney R, Warner J, Iliffe S, van Haselen R, Griffin M, Fisher P. The Hawthorne effect: a randomised, controlled trial. *BMC Medical Research Methodology* 2007;7:30.

189 Armitage P, Berry G, Matthews JNS (eds) *Statistical Methods in Medical Research,* 4th edn. Oxford: Blackwell Science, 2002.

190 Moncrieff J, Wessely S. Active placebos in antidepressant trials. *British Journal of Psychiatry* 1998;173:88.

191 Moncrieff J. A comparison of antidepressant trials using active and inert placebos. *International Journal of Methods in Psychiatric Research* 2003;12: 117–27.

192 Moncrieff J, Wessely S, Hardy R. Active placebos versus antidepressants for depression. *Cochrane Database of Systematic Reviews* 2004;(1):CD003012.

193 Tuteur W. The double blind method: its pitfalls and fallacies. *American Journal of Psychiatry* 1958;114:921–2.

194 Rosenthal R, Lawson R. A longitudinal study of the effects of experimenter bias on the operant learning of laboratory rats. *Journal of Psychiatric Research* 1964;69:61–72.

195 Eisenach JC, Lindner MD. Did experimenter bias conceal the efficacy of spinal opioids in previous studies with the spinal nerve ligation model of neuropathic pain? *Anesthesiology* 2004;100:765–7.

196 Berkson J, Magath T, Hurn M. The error of estimate of the blood cell count as made with the hmocytometer. *American Journal of Physiology* 1939;128:309–23.

197 Urbach P. Randomization and the design of experiments. *Philosophy of Science* 1985;52:256–73.

198 Fisher RA. *The Design of Experiments,* 4th edn. Edinburgh: Oliver & Boyd, 1947.

199 Lonn EM, Yusuf S. Is there a role for antioxidant vitamins in the prevention of cardiovascular diseases? An update on epidemiological and clinical trials data. *Canadian Journal of Cardiology* 1997;13:957–65.

200 Patterson RE, White E, Kristal AR, Neuhouser ML, Potter JD. Vitamin supplements and cancer risk: the epidemiologic evidence. *Cancer Causes and Control* 1997;8:786–802.

201 Farley SM, Libanati CR, Odvina CV *et al.* Efficacy of long-term fluoride and calcium therapy in correcting the deficit of spinal bone density in osteoporosis. *Journal of Clinical Epidemiology* 1989;42:1067–74.

202 Riggs BL, Hodgson SF, O'Fallon WM *et al.* Effect of fluoride treatment on the fracture rate in postmenopausal women with osteoporosis. *New England Journal of Medicine.* 1990;322:802–9.

203 Knekt P, Reunanen A, Jarvinen R, Seppanen R, Heliovaara M, Aromaa A. Antioxidant vitamin intake and coronary mortality in a longitudinal population study. *American Journal of Epidemiology* 1994;139:1180–9.

204 Yusuf S, Dagenais G, Pogue J, Bosch J, Sleight P. Vitamin E supplementation and cardiovascular events in high-risk patients. The Heart Outcomes Prevention Evaluation Study Investigators. *New England Journal of Medicine* 2000;342:154–60.

205 Cotroneo AR, Di Stasi C, Cina A, Di Gregorio F. Venous interruption as prophylaxis of pulmonary embolism: vena cava filters. *Rays* 1996;21:461–80.

206 Decousus H, Leizorovicz A, Parent F *et al.* A clinical trial of vena caval filters in the prevention of pulmonary embolism in patients with proximal deep-vein thrombosis. *New England Journal of Medicine* 1998;338:409–15.

207 Petitti DB. Coronary heart disease and estrogen replacement therapy. Can compliance bias explain the results of observational studies? *Annals of Epidemiology* 1994;4:115–18.

208 Finucane FF, Madans JH, Bush TL, Wolf PH, Kleinman JC. Decreased risk of stroke among postmenopausal hormone users. Results from a national cohort. *Archives of Internal Medicine* 1993;153:73–9.

209 Rossouw JE, Anderson GL, Prentice RL *et al.* Risks and benefits of estrogen plus progestin in healthy postmenopausal women: principal results from the Women's Health Initiative randomized controlled trial. *Journal of the American Medical Association* 2002;288:321–33.

210 Wassertheil-Smoller S, Hendrix SL, Limacher M *et al.* Effect of estrogen plus progestin on stroke in postmenopausal women: the Women's Health Initiative: a randomized trial. *Journal of the American Medical Association* 2003;289:2673–84.

211 Gøtzsche PC, Olsen O. Is screening for breast cancer with mammography justifiable? *Lancet* 2000;355:129–34.

212 Kunz R, Khan KS, Neumayer HH. Observational studies and randomized trials. *New England Journal of Medicine* 2000;343:1194–5; author reply 6–7.

213 Ioannidis JP. Contradicted and initially stronger effects in highly cited clinical research. *Journal of the American Medical Association* 2005;294:218–28.

214 Ziegler EJ, Fisher CJ Jr, Sprung CL *et al.* Treatment of gram-negative bacteremia and septic shock with HA-1A human monoclonal antibody against endotoxin. A randomized, double-blind, placebo-controlled trial. *New England Journal of Medicine* 1991;324:429–36.

215 McCloskey RV, Straube RC, Sanders C, Smith SM, Smith CR. Treatment of septic shock with human monoclonal antibody HA-1A. A randomized, double-blind, placebo-controlled trial. *Annals of Internal Medicine* 1994;121:1–5.

216 Keen HI, Pile K, Hill CL. The prevalence of underpowered randomized clinical trials in rheumatology. *Journal of Rheumatology* 2005;32:2083–8.

217 Schulz KF, Chalmers I, Hayes RJ, Altman DG. Empirical evidence of bias. Dimensions of methodological quality associated with estimates of treatment effects in controlled trials. *Journal of the American Medical Association* 1995;273:408–12.

218 Viera AJ, Bangdiwala SI. Eliminating bias in randomized controlled trials: importance of allocation concealment and masking. *Family Medicine* 2007;39:132–7.

219 Wood L, Egger M, Gluud LL *et al.* Empirical evidence of bias in treatment effect estimates in controlled trials with different interventions and outcomes: meta-epidemiological study. *British Medical Journal* 2008;336:601–5.

220 Crossley NA, Sena E, Goehler J *et al.* Empirical evidence of bias in the design of experimental stroke studies: a metaepidemiologic approach. *Stroke* 2008;39:929–34.

221 Schulz KF, Chalmers I, Altman DG. The landscape and lexicon of blinding in randomized trials. *Annals of Internal Medicine* 2002;136:254–9.

222 Schulz KF, Grimes DA. Blinding in randomised trials: hiding who got what. *Lancet* 2002;359:696–700.

223 Bhardwaj SS, Camacho F, Derrow A, Fleischer AB Jr, Feldman SR. Statistical significance and clinical relevance: the importance of power in clinical trials in dermatology. *Archives of Dermatology* 2004;140:1520–3.

224 Luus HG, Muller FO, Meyer BH. Statistical significance versus clinical relevance. Part I. The essential role of the power of a statistical test. *South African Medical Journal.* 1989;76:568–70.

225 Sierevelt IN, van Oldenrijk J, Poolman RW. Is statistical significance clinically important? A guide to judge the clinical relevance of study findings. *Journal of Long-term Effects of Medical Implants* 2007;17:173–9.

226 Barbui C, Cipriani A. Publication bias in systematic reviews. *Archives of General Psychiatry* 2007;64:868.

227 Gluud LL. Unravelling industry bias in clinical trials. *Pain* 2006;121:175–6.

228 Procopio M. The multiple outcomes bias in antidepressants research. *Medical Hypotheses* 2005;65:395–9.

229 Smith GD, Ebrahim S. Data dredging, bias, or confounding. *British Medical Journal* 2002;325:1437–8.

230 Altman D, Schulz K, Moher D *et al.* The revised CONSORT statement for reporting randomized trials: explanation and elaboration. *Annals of Internal Medicine* 2001;134:663–94.

231 Altman DG. Poor-quality medical research: what can journals do? *Journal of the American Medical Association* 2002;287:2765–7.

232 Ioannidis JP. Why most published research findings are false. *PLoS Med* 2005;2(8):e124.

233 Cartwright N. What is this thing called efficacy. In: Mantzavinos C (ed.) *Philosophy of the Social Sciences Philosophical Theory and Scientific Practice.* Cambridge: Cambridge University Press, 2009.

234 Vandenbroucke JP, von Elm E, Altman DG *et al.* Strengthening the Reporting of Observational Studies in Epidemiology (STROBE): explanation and elaboration. *PLoS Med* 2007;4(10):e297.

235 Vist GE, Bryant D, Somerville L, Birminghem T, Oxman AD. Outcomes of patients who participate in randomized controlled trials compared to similar patients receiving similar interventions who do not participate. *Cochrane Database of Systematic Reviews* 2008;(3):MR000009.

236 Vist GE, Hagen KB, Devereaux PJ, Bryant D, Kristoffersen DT, Oxman AD. Outcomes of patients who participate in randomised controlled trials compared to similar patients receiving similar interventions who do not participate. *Cochrane Database of Systematic Reviews* 2007;(2):MR000009.

237 Vist GE, Hagen KB, Devereaux PJ, Bryant D, Kristoffersen DT, Oxman AD. Systematic review to determine whether participation in a trial influences outcome. *British Medical Journal* 2005;330:1175.

238 Golomb B, Erickson LC, Koperski S, Sack D, Enkin M, Howick J. What's in placebos: who knows? Analysis of randomized, controlled trials. *Annals of Internal Medicine* 2010;153(8):532–5.

239 Arroll B, Macgillivray S, Ogston S *et al.* Efficacy and tolerability of tricyclic antidepressants and SSRIs compared with placebo for treatment of depression in primary care: a meta-analysis. *Annals of Family Medicine* 2005;3: 449–56.

240 Williams JW Jr, Mulrow CD, Chiquette E, Noel PH, Aguilar C, Cornell J. A systematic review of newer pharmacotherapies for depression in adults: evidence report summary. *Annals of Internal Medicine* 2000;132:743–56.

241 Nemeroff CB, Entsuah R, Benattia I, Demitrack M, Sloan DM, Thase ME. Comprehensive analysis of remission (COMPARE) with venlafaxine versus SSRIs. *Biological Psychiatry* 2008;63:424–34.

242 Whittington CJ, Kendall T, Fonagy P, Cottrell D, Cotgrove A, Boddington E. Selective serotonin reuptake inhibitors in childhood depression: systematic review of published versus unpublished data. *Lancet* 2004;363:1341–5.

243 Perlis RH, Perlis CS, Wu Y, Hwang C, Joseph M, Nierenberg AA. Industry sponsorship and financial conflict of interest in the reporting of clinical trials in psychiatry. *American Journal of Psychiatry* 2005;162:1957–60.

244 National Institutes of Health. Available at www.clinicaltrials.gov [updated July 2006; accessed November 23, 2006]

245 Gaudilliere JP. Beyond one-case statistics: mathematics, medicine, and the management of health and disease in the postwar era. In: Bottazzini U, Dalmedico AD (eds) *Changing Images in Mathematics: From the French Revolution to the New Millenium*. London: Routledge, 2001.

246 Marks HM. *The Progress of Experiment: Science and Therapeutic Reform in the United States 1900–1990*. Cambridge: Cambridge University Press, 1997.

247 Matthews JR. *Quantification and the Quest for Medical Certainty*. Princeton: Princeton University Press, 1995.

248 Chalmers I. Statistical theory was not the reason that randomization was used in the British Medical Research Council's clinical trial of streptomycin for pulmonary tuberculosis. In: Jorland G, Opinel A, Weisz G (eds) *Body*

Counts: Medical Quantification in Historical and Sociological Perspectives. Montreal: McGill-Queens University Press, 2005, pp. 309–34.

249 Lasagna L. The controlled clinical trial: theory and practice. *Journal of Chronic Diseases* 1955;1:353–67.

250 Yoshioka A. Use of randomisation in the Medical Research Council's clinical trial of streptomycin in pulmonary tuberculosis in the 1940s. *British Medical Journal* 1998;317:1220–3.

251 Cartwright N. *Nature's Capacities and their Measurement*. Oxford: Clarendon Press, 1989.

252 Papineau D. The virtues of randomization. *British Journal for the Philosophy of Science* 1994;45:437–50.

253 Pearl J. *Causality: Models, Reasoning, and Inference*. Cambridge: Cambridge University Press, 2000.

254 "Guidance for Industry, Investigators, and Reviewers". Food and Drug Administration. January 2006. http://www.fda.gov/downloads/Drugs/Guidance ComplianceRegulatoryInformation/Guidances/ucm078933.pdf, accessed 21 December 2010.

255 Altman DG, Schulz KF, Moher D *et al*. The revised CONSORT statement for reporting randomized trials: explanation and elaboration. *Annals of Internal Medicine* 2001;134:663–94.

256 Guyatt G, Oxman A, Kunz R, Vist GE, Falck-Ytter Y, Schünemann HJ. Rating quality of evidence and strength of recommendation: What is "quality of evidence" and why is it important to clinicians? *British Medical Journal* 2008;336:995–8.

257 Greenhalgh T. *How to Read a Paper: the Basics of Evidence-based Medicine*, 3rd edn. Malden, MA: BMJ Books/Blackwell Publishing, 2006.

258 Kaptchuk TJ, Kelley JM, Conboy LA *et al*. Components of placebo effect: randomised controlled trial in patients with irritable bowel syndrome. *British Medical Journal* 2008;336:999–1003.

259 Ney PG, Collins C, Spensor C. Double blind: double talk or are there ways to do better research. *Medical Hypotheses* 1986;21:119–26.

260 Kaptchuk TJ. Intentional ignorance: a history of blind assessment and placebo controls in medicine. *Bulletin of the History of Medicine* 1998;72: 389–433.

261 Schulz KF, Altman DG, Moher D. CONSORT 2010 statement: updated guidelines for reporting parallel group randomised trials. *PLoS Med* 2010;7(3): e1000251.

262 Colloca L, Lopiano L, Lanotte M, Benedetti F. Overt versus covert treatment for pain, anxiety, and Parkinson's disease. *Lancet Neurology* 2004;3:679–84.

263 Kirsch I. Conditioning, expectancy, and the placebo effect: comment on Stewart-Williams and Podd (2004). *Psychological Bulletin* 2004;130:341–3; discussion 4–5.

264 Moerman DE, Jonas WB. Deconstructing the placebo effect and finding the meaning response. *Annals of Internal Medicine* 2002;136:471–6.

265 Rosenthal R, Jacobson LF. *Pygmalion in the Classroom: Teacher Expectation and Pupils' Intellectual Development*. New York: Irvington Publishers, 1992.

266 Fergusson D, Glass KC, Waring D, Shapiro S. Turning a blind eye: the success of blinding reported in a random sample of randomised, placebo controlled trials. *British Medical Journal* 2004;328:432.

267 Hrobjartsson A, Forfang E, Haahr MT, Als-Nielsen B, Brorson S. Blinded trials taken to the test: an analysis of randomized clinical trials that report tests for the success of blinding. *International Journal of Epidemiology* 2007;36:654–63.

268 Edward SJ, Stevens AJ, Braunholtz DA, Lilford RJ, Swift T. The ethics of placebo-controlled trials: a comparison of inert and active placebo controls. *World Journal of Surgery* 2005;29:610–14.

269 Kirsch I. Yes, there is a placebo effect, but is there a powerful antidepressant effect? *Prevention and Treatment* 2002;5(22).

270 Kemp AS, Schooler NR, Kalali AH *et al.* What is causing the reduced drug–placebo difference in recent schizophrenia clinical trials and what can be done about it? *Schizophrenia Bulletin* 2010;36:504–9.

271 Benedetti F, Pollo A, Lopiano L, Lanotte M, Vighetti S, Rainero I. Conscious expectation and unconscious conditioning in analgesic, motor, and hormonal placebo/nocebo responses. *Journal of Neuroscience* 2003;23:4315–23.

272 Golomb B. When are medication side effects due to the nocebo phenomenon? *Journal of the American Medical Association* 2002;287:2502–3.

273 Johansen O, Brox J, Flaten MA. Placebo and nocebo responses, cortisol, and circulating beta-endorphin. *Psychosomatic Medicine* 2003;65:786–90.

274 Kong J, Gollub RL, Polich G *et al.* A functional magnetic resonance imaging study on the neural mechanisms of hyperalgesic nocebo effect. *Journal of Neuroscience* 2008;28:13354–62.

275 Freed CR, Greene PE, Breeze RE *et al.* Transplantation of embryonic dopamine neurons for severe Parkinson's disease. *New England Journal of Medicine* 2001;344:710–19.

276 Moseley JB, O'Malley K, Petersen NJ *et al.* A controlled trial of arthroscopic surgery for osteoarthritis of the knee. *New England Journal of Medicine* 2002;347:81–8.

277 Connolly SJ, Sheldon R, Thorpe KE *et al.* Pacemaker therapy for prevention of syncope in patients with recurrent severe vasovagal syncope. Second Vasovagal Pacemaker Study (VPS II): a randomized trial. *Journal of the American Medical Association* 2003;289:2224–9.

278 Olanow CW, Goetz CG, Kordower JH *et al.* A double-blind controlled trial of bilateral fetal nigral transplantation in Parkinson's disease. *Annals of Neurology* 2003;54:403–14.

279 Gragoudas ES, Adamis AP, Cunningham ET Jr, Feinsod M, Guyer DR. Pegaptanib for neovascular age-related macular degeneration. *New England Journal of Medicine* 2004;351:2805–16.

280 Heckerling PS. Placebo surgery research: a blinding imperative. *Journal of Clinical Epidemiology* 2006;59:876–80.

281 Katz RD, Taylor JA, Rosson GD, Brown PR, Singh NK. Robotics in plastic and reconstructive surgery: use of a telemanipulator slave robot to perform microvascular anastomoses. *Journal of Reconstructive Microsurgery* 2006;22:53–7.

282 Worn H. Computer- and robot-aided head surgery. *Acta Neurochirurgica Supplementum* 2006;98:51–61.

283 Diks J, Nio D, Jongkind V, Cuesta MA, Rauwerda JA, Wisselink W. Robot-assisted laparoscopic surgery of the infrarenal aorta: the early learning curve. *Surgical Endoscopy* 2007;21:1760–3.

284 Suzuki N, Hattori A, Suzuki S, Otake Y. Development of a surgical robot system for endovascular surgery with augmented reality function. *Studies in Health Technology and Informatics* 2007;125:460–3.

285 Sackett D. Commentary. Measuring the success of blinding in RCTs: don't, must, can't, or needn't? *International Journal of Epidemiology* 2007;36:664–5.

286 Schulz KF, Altman DG, Moher D, Fergusson D. CONSORT 2010 changes and testing blindness in RCTs. *Lancet* 2010;375:1144–6.

287 Shapiro S. Widening the field of vision. *British Medical Journal*. 2004 (http://www.bmj.com/content/328/7437/432/reply), accessed 21 December 2010.

288 de Craen AJ, Roos PJ, Leonard de Vries A, Kleijnen J. Effect of colour of drugs: systematic review of perceived effect of drugs and of their effectiveness. *British Medical Journal* 1996;313:1624–6.

289 Golomb BA. Paradox of placebo effect. *Nature* 1995;375:530.

290 Shapiro A, Morris LA. The placebo effect in medical and psychological therapies. In: Garfield SL, Bergin AE (eds) *Handbook of Psychotherapy and Behavioral Change: An Empirical Analysis*. New York: John Wiley & Sons, 1978, pp. 369–410.

291 Grünbaum A. The placebo concept in medicine and psychiatry. *Psychological Medicine* 1986;16:19–38.

292 Benedetti F, Amanzio M. The neurobiology of placebo analgesia: from endogenous opioids to cholecystokinin. *Progress in Neurobiology* 1997;52: 109–25.

293 Wager TD, Rilling JK, Smith EE *et al*. Placebo-induced changes in FMRI in the anticipation and experience of pain. *Science* 2004;303:1162–7.

294 Petrovic P, Kalso E, Petersson KM, Ingvar M. Placebo and opioid analgesia: imaging a shared neuronal network. *Science* 2002;295:1737–40.

295 Bingel U, Lorenz J, Schoell E, Weiller C, Buchel C. Mechanisms of placebo analgesia: rACC recruitment of a subcortical antinociceptive network. *Pain* 2006;120:8–15.

296 Oken BS. Placebo effects: clinical aspects and neurobiology. *Brain* 2008;131:2812–23.

297 Kong J, Kaptchuk TJ, Polich G, Kirsch I, Gollub RL. Placebo analgesia: findings from brain imaging studies and emerging hypotheses. *Reviews in the Neurosciences* 2007;18:173–90.

298 Craggs JG, Price DD, Verne GN, Perlstein WM, Robinson MM. Functional brain interactions that serve cognitive-affective processing during pain and placebo analgesia. *Neuroimage* 2007;38:720–9.

299 Moerman DE. General medical effectiveness and human biology: placebo effects in the treatment of ulcer disease. *Medical Anthropology Quarterly* 1983;14:13–16.

300 Evans D. *Placebo: The Belief Effect*. London: Harper Collins, 2003.

301 Golomb B, Erickson LC, Koperski S, Sack D, Enkin M, Howick J. What's in placebos: who knows? Analysis of randomized, controlled trials. *Annals of Internal Medicine* 2010;153(8):532–5.

302 Howick J. Escaping from placebo prison. *British Medical Journal* 2009;338: b1898.

303 Nunn R. It's time to put the placebo out of its misery. *British Medical Journal* 2009;338:1015.

304 Park LC, Covi L. Nonblind placebo trial: an exploration of neurotic patients' responses to placebo when its inert content is disclosed. *Archives of General Psychiatry* 1965;12:36–45.

305 Paul IM, Beiler J, McMonagle A, Shaffer ML, Duda L, Berlin CM Jr. Effect of honey, dextromethorphan, and no treatment on nocturnal cough and sleep quality for coughing children and their parents. *Archives of Pediatrics and Adolescent Medicine* 2007;161:1140–6.

306 Eccles R. Mechanisms of the placebo effect of sweet cough syrups. *Respiratory Physiology and Neurobiology* 2006;152:340–8.

307 Brown BS, Payne T, Kim C, Moore G, Krebs P, Martin W. Chronic response of rat brain norepinephrine and serotonin levels to endurance training. *Journal of Applied Physiology: Respiratory, Environmental and Exercise Physiology* 1979;46:19–23.

308 Koch G, Johansson U, Arvidsson E. Radioenzymatic determination of epine-phrine, norepinephrine, and dopamine in 0.1 mL plasma samples: plasma catecholamine response to submaximal and near maximal exercise. *Journal of Clinical Chemistry and Clinical Biochemistry* 1980;18:367–72.

309 McCann IL, Holmes DS. Influence of aerobic exercise on depression. *Journal of Personality and Social Psychology* 1984;46:1142–7.

310 Dunn AL, Trivedi MH, Kampert JB, Clark CG, Chambliss HO. The DOSE study: a clinical trial to examine efficacy and dose response of exercise as treatment for depression. *Controlled Clinical Trials* 2002;23:584–603.

311 Dunn AL, Trivedi MH, Kampert JB, Clark CG, Chambliss HO. Exercise treatment for depression: efficacy and dose response. *American Journal of Preventive Medicine* 2005;28:1–8.

312 Hamilton M. Development of a rating scale for primary depressive illness. *British Journal of Social and Clinical Psychology* 1967;6:278–96.

313 Woolery A, Myers H, Sternlieb B, Zeltzer L. A yoga intervention for young adults with elevated symptoms of depression. *Alternative Therapies in Health and Medicine* 2004;10:60–3.

314 Choate JK, Kato K, Mohan RM. Exercise training enhances relaxation of the isolated guinea-pig saphenous artery in response to acetylcholine. *Experimental Physiology* 2000;85:103–8.

315 Streitberger K, Kleinhenz J. Introducing a placebo needle into acupuncture research. *Lancet* 1998;352:364–5.

316 Kleinhenz J, Streitberger K, Windeler J, Gussbacher A, Mavridis G, Martin E. Randomised clinical trial comparing the effects of acupuncture and a newly designed placebo needle in rotator cuff tendinitis. *Pain* 1999;83: 235–41.

317 White P, Lewith G, Hopwood V, Prescott P. The placebo needle, is it a valid and convincing placebo for use in acupuncture trials? A randomised, single-blind, cross-over pilot trial. *Pain* 2003;106:401–9.

318 Birch S. Comment on sham device v inert pill: randomised controlled trial of two placebo treatments. Available at www.bmj.com [accessed February 9, 2006]

319 Birch S. Yes, let's get real: what the placebo isn't. Available at www.bmj.com [accessed March 10, 2006]

320 Lewith GT, White A. A true placebo? Available at www.bmj.com [accessed February 3, 2006]

321 Lewith GT. Re: A plastic eagle feather. Available at www.bmj.com [accessed February 8, 2006]

322 Li SM, Costi JM, Teixeira JE. Sham acupuncture is not a placebo. *Archives of Internal Medicine* 2008;168:1011; author reply 2.

323 Heyland SJ, Moorey J. Doctor–patient interaction is not an element of the placebo effect. Available at www.bmj.com/cgi/eletters/bmj.39524.439618.25 v1#195429 [accessed July 21, 2010]

324 Kaptchuk TJ, Stason WB, Davis RB *et al.* Sham device v inert pill: randomised controlled trial of two placebo treatments. *British Medical Journal* 2006;332:391–7.

325 Haake M, Muller HH, Schade-Brittinger C *et al.* German Acupuncture Trials (GERAC) for chronic low back pain: randomized, multicenter, blinded, parallel-group trial with 3 groups. *Archives of Internal Medicine* 2007;167:1892–8.

326 Sprott H, Gay RE, Michel BA, Gay S. Influence of ibuprofen-arginine on serum levels of nitric oxide metabolites in patients with chronic low back pain: a single-blind, placebo controlled pilot trial (ISRCTN18723747). *Journal of Rheumatology* 2006;33:2515–18.

327 Coats TL, Borenstein DG, Nangia NK, Brown MT. Effects of valdecoxib in the treatment of chronic low back pain: results of a randomized, placebo-controlled trial. *Clinical Therapeutics* 2004;26:1249–60.

328 Roelofs PD, Deyo RA, Koes BW, Scholten RJ, van Tulder MW. Nonsteroidal anti-inflammatory drugs for low back pain: an updated cochrane review. *Spine* 2008;33:1766–74.

329 Lee A, Done ML. Stimulation of the wrist acupuncture point P6 for preventing postoperative nausea and vomiting. *Cochrane Database of Systematic Reviews.* 2004;(3):CD003281.

330 Agarwal A, Ranjan R, Dhiraaj S, Lakra A, Kumar M, Singh U. Acupressure for prevention of pre-operative anxiety: a prospective, randomised, placebo controlled study. *Anaesthesia* 2005;60:978–81.

331 Ezzo J, Streitberger K, Schneider A. Cochrane systematic reviews examine P6 acupuncture-point stimulation for nausea and vomiting. *Journal of Alternative and Complementary Medicine* 2006;12:489–95.

332 Paterson C, Dieppe P. Characteristic and incidental (placebo) effects in complex interventions such as acupuncture. *British Medical Journal* 2005;330:1202–5.

333 Howick J. *Philosophical Issues in Evidence-based Medicine: Evaluating the Epistemological Role of Double Blinding and Placebo Controls.* London: London School of Economics, 2008.

334 Temple R, Ellenberg SS. Placebo-controlled trials and active-control trials in the evaluation of new treatments. Part 1: ethical and scientific issues. *Annals of Internal Medicine* 2000;133:455–63.

335 Ellenberg SS, Temple R. Placebo-controlled trials and active-control trials in the evaluation of new treatments. Part 2: practical issues and specific cases. *Annals of Internal Medicine* 2000;133:464–70.

336 International Conference on Harmonization. Harmonized Tripartite Guideline. Choice of Control Group and Related Issues in Clinical Trials. E10. Geneva: Centre for Biologics Evaluation and Research, 2000.

337 World Medical Association. *The Declaration of Helsinki*. Seoul: WMA, 2008. Available at www.wma.net/e/ [updated October 2008, accessed July 7, 2009]

338 Miller FG, Brody H. What makes placebo-controlled trials unethical? *American Journal of Bioethics* 2002;2:3–9.

339 World Medical Association. World Medical Association International Code of Medical Ethics. *Policy*. London: WMA, 1949.

340 General Medical Council. *Good Medical Practice. The Duties of a Doctor Registered with the General Medical Council.* London: GMC, 2006.

341 Lasagna L. Hippocratic Oath, modern version. Available at www.pbs.org/wgbh/nova/doctors/oath_modern.html [accessed February 9, 2009]

342 Altman DG. Statistics and ethics in medical research. Misuse of statistics is unethical. *British Medical Journal* 1980;281:1182–4.

343 Emanuel EJ, Wendler D, Grady C. What makes clinical research ethical? *Journal of the American Medical Association* 2000;283:2701–11.

344 Halpern SD, Karlawish JH, Berlin JA. The continuing unethical conduct of underpowered clinical trials. *Journal of the American Medical Association* 2002;288:358–62.

345 Council for International Organizations of Medical Sciences. Geneva: CIOMS, 1993. www.cioms.ch [accessed December 21, 2010].

346 Council for International Organizations of Medical Sciences. *International Ethical Guidelines for Biomedical Research Involving Human Subjects.* Geneva: CIOMS, 1993.

347 Hwang IK, Morikawa T. Design issues in noninferiority/equivalence trials. *Drug Information Journal* 1999;33:1205–18.

348 Shapiro A, Shapiro E. The placebo. Is it much ado about nothing? In: Harrington A (ed.) *The Placebo Effect: An Interdisciplinary Exploration.* Harvard University Press, Cambridge, Massachusetts, 1997.

349 Wootton D. *Bad Medicine: Doctors Doing Harm Since Hippocrates.* Oxford: Oxford University Press, 2006.

350 Echt DS, Liebson PR, Mitchell LB *et al.* Mortality and morbidity in patients receiving encainide, flecainide, or placebo. The Cardiac Arrhythmia Suppression Trial. *New England Journal of Medicine* 1991;324:781–8.

351 Takala J, Ruokonen E, Webster NR *et al.* Increased mortality associated with growth hormone treatment in critically ill adults. *New England Journal of Medicine* 1999;341:785–92.

352 Hayes MA, Timmins AC, Yau EH, Palazzo M, Hinds CJ, Watson D. Elevation of systemic oxygen delivery in the treatment of critically ill patients. *New England Journal of Medicine* 1994;330:1717–22.

353 Herbert PC, Wells G, Blajchman MA. A multicenter, randomized, controlled clinical trial of transfusion requirements in critical care. New *England Journal of Medicine* 1999;340:409–17.

354 ALLHAT Collaborative Research Group. Major cardiovascular events in hypertensive patients randomized to doxazosin vs chlorthalidone: the antihypertensive and lipid-lowering treatment to prevent heart attack trial (ALLHAT). *Journal of the American Medical Association* 2000;283:1967–75.

355 Dwyer T, Ponsonby AL. Sudden infant death syndrome: after the "back to sleep" campaign. *British Medical Journal* 1996;313:180–1.

356 Ebell MH, Siwek J, Weiss BD *et al*. Strength of recommendation taxonomy (SORT): a patient-centered approach to grading evidence in the medical literature. *American Family Physician* 2004;69:548–56.

357 Moerman DE. Cultural variations in the placebo effect: ulcers, anxiety, and blood pressure. *Medical Anthropology Quarterly* 2000;14:51–72.

358 Patel SM, Stason WB, Legedza A *et al*. The placebo effect in irritable bowel syndrome trials: a meta-analysis. *Neurogastroenterology and Motility* 2005;17:332–40.

359 Smith R. Where is the wisdom . . . ? *British Medical Journal* 1991;303:798–9.

360 Ellis J, Mulligan I, Rowe J, Sackett DL. Inpatient general medicine is evidence based. A-Team, Nuffield Department of Clinical Medicine. *Lancet* 1995;346:407–10.

361 Gill P, Dowell AC, Neal RD, Smith N, Heywood P, Wilson AE. Evidence based general practice: a retrospective study of interventions in one training practice. *British Medical Journal* 1996;312:819–21.

362 Imrie R, Ramey DW. The evidence for evidence-based medicine. *Complementary Therapies in Medicine* 2000;8:123–6.

363 Dickersin K. The existence of publication bias and risk factors for its occurrence. *Journal of the American Medical Association* 1990;263:1385–9.

364 Davidson RA. Source of funding and outcome of clinical trials. *Journal of General Internal Medicine* 1986;1:155–8.

365 Kirsch I, Deacon BJ, Huedo-Medina TB, Scoboria A, Moore TJ, Johnson BT. Initial severity and antidepressant benefits: a meta-analysis of data submitted to the Food and Drug Administration. *PLoS Med* 2008;5(2):e45.

366 The EC/IC Bypass Study Group. Failure of extracranial–intracranial arterial bypass to reduce the risk of ischemic stroke. Results of an international randomized trial. *New England Journal of Medicine* 1985;313:1191–200.

367 Sackett DL, Spitzer WO, Gent M, Roberts RS. The Burlington randomized trial of the nurse practitioner: health outcomes of patients. *Annals of Internal Medicine* 1974;80:137–42.

368 Morgan SG, Bassett KL, Wright JM *et al*. "Breakthrough" drugs and growth in expenditure on prescription drugs in Canada. *British Medical Journal* 2005;331:815–16.

369 Senn SJ. Active control equivalence studies. In: Everitt BS, Palmer CR (eds) *Encyclopaedic Companion to Medical Statistics*. London: Hodder Arnold, 2005, pp. 19–22.

370 Piaggio G, Elbourne DR, Altman DG, Pocock SJ, Evans SJ. Reporting of noninferiority and equivalence randomized trials: an extension of the

CONSORT statement. *Journal of the American Medical Association* 2006;295: 1152–60.

371 Garattini S, Bertele V. Non-inferiority trials are unethical because they disregard patients' interests. *Lancet* 2007;370:1875–7.

372 Goff DC, Lamberti JS, Leon AC *et al.* A placebo-controlled add-on trial of the Ampakine, CX516, for cognitive deficits in schizophrenia. *Neuropsychopharmacology* 2008;33:465–72.

373 Dunnett CW, Gent M. Significance testing to establish equivalence between treatments, with special reference to data in the form of 2×2 tables. *Biometrics* 1977;33:593–602.

374 Blackwelder WC. "Proving the null hypothesis" in clinical trials. *Controlled Clinical Trials* 1982;3:345–53.

375 Gomberg-Maitland M, Frison L, Halperin JL. Active-control clinical trials to establish equivalence or noninferiority: methodological and statistical concepts linked to quality. *American Heart Journal* 2003;146:398–403.

376 Senn SJ. *Statistical Issues in Drug Development*, 2nd edn. Hoboken, NJ: Wiley, 2007.

377 Kleijnen J, de Craen AJ, van Everdingen J, Krol L. Placebo effect in double-blind clinical trials: a review of interactions with medications. *Lancet* 1994;344:1347–9.

378 Kirsch I. Are drug and placebo effects in depression additive? *Biological Psychiatry* 2000;47:733–5.

379 Kaptchuk TJ. The double-blind, randomized, placebo-controlled trial: gold standard or golden calf? *Journal of Clinical Epidemiology* 2001;54:541–9.

380 Hughes JR, Gulliver SB, Amori G, Mireault GC, Fenwick JF. Effect of instructions and nicotine on smoking cessation, withdrawal symptoms and self-administration of nicotine gum. *Psychopharmacology (Berl)* 1989;99:486–91.

381 Levine JD, Gordon NC. Influence of the method of drug administration on analgesic response. *Nature* 1984;312:755–6.

382 Mitchell SH, Laurent CL, de Wit H. Interaction of expectancy and the pharmacological effects of D-amphetamine: subjective effects and self-administration. *Psychopharmacology (Berl)* 1996;125:371–8.

383 Ross DF, Krugman AD, Lyerly SB, Clyde DJ. Drugs and placebos: a model design. *Psychological Reports* 1962;10:383–92.

384 Freud S, Strachey J, Freud A, Richards A. *The Standard Edition of the Complete Psychological Works of Sigmund Freud*, Vol. 24, Indexes and bibliographies. London: Vintage, 2001.

385 Aronson JK. Concentration–effect and dose–response relations in clinical pharmacology. *British Journal of Clinical Pharmacology* 2007;63:255–7.

386 ter Riet G, de Craen AJ, de Boer A, Kessels AG. Is placebo analgesia mediated by endogenous opioids? A systematic review. *Pain* 1998;76:273–5.

387 Anderson JA. The ethics and science of placebo-controlled trials: assay sensitivity and the Duhem–Quine thesis. *Journal of Medicine and Philosophy* 2006;31:65–81.

388 Hume D, Norton DF, Norton MJ. *A Treatise of Human Nature*. Oxford: Oxford University Press, 2000.

389 Bacon F. *Novum Organum*. Devey J (ed.) New York: P.F. Collier, 1902.

390 Bechtel W, Abrahamsen A. Explanation: a mechanist alternative. *Studies in the History and Philosophy of Biological and Biomedical Sciences* 2005;36:421–41.
391 Bechtel W. *Discovering Cell Mechanisms: The Creation of Modern Cell Biology*. New York: Cambridge University Press, 2006.
392 Bogen J. Regularities and causality; generalizations and causal explanations. *Studies in the History and Philosophy of Biological and Biomedical Sciences* 2005;36:197–420.
393 Bogen J. Causally productive activities. *Studies in the History and Philosophy of Biological and Biomedical Sciences* 2008;39:112–23.
394 Craver CF. Role functions, mechanisms, and hierarchy. *Philosophy of Science* 2001;68:53–74.
395 Craver CF. Beyond reduction: mechanisms, multifield integration, and the unity of neuroscience. *Studies in the History and Philosophy of Biological and Biomedical Sciences* 2005;36:373–97.
396 Darden L. Discovering mechanisms: a computational philosophy of science perspective. In: Jantke KP, Shinohara A (eds) *Discovery Science*. New York: Springer, 2001.
397 Darden L. *Reasoning in Biological Discoveries: Mechanisms, Interfield Relations, and Anomaly Resolution*. New York: Cambridge University Press, 2006.
398 Darden L. Thinking again about biological mechanisms. *Philosophy of Science* 2008;75:958–69.
399 Glennan SS. Mechanisms and the nature of causation. *Erkentnis* 1996;44: 49–71.
400 Glennan SS. Rethinking mechanistic explanation. *Philosophy of Science* 2002;69:S342–S353.
401 Machamer P, Darden L, Craver CF. Thinking about mechanisms. *Philosophy of Science* 2000;67:1–25.
402 Machamer P. Activities and causation: the metaphysics and epistemology of mechanisms. *International Studies in the Philosophy of Science* 2004;18:27–39.
403 Russo F, Williamson J. Interpreting causality in the health sciences. *International Studies in the Philosophy of Science* 2007;21:1157–70.
404 Gillies D. The Russo–Williamson thesis and the question of whether smoking causes heart disease. forthcoming.
405 Howick J. Double-blinding: the benefits and risks of being kept in the dark. In: Fennell D (ed.) *Contingency and Dissent in Science*. Technical Report 03/08. London: Contingency And Dissent in Science Project, 2008.
406 Psillos S. A glimpse of the secret connexion: harmonizing mechanisms with counterfactuals. *Perspectives on Science* 2004;12:288–319.
407 Bayes de Luna A, Coumel P, Leclercq JF. Ambulatory sudden cardiac death: mechanisms of production of fatal arrhythmia on the basis of data from 157 cases. *American Heart Journal* 1989;117:151–9.
408 Huikuri HV, Castellanos A, Myerburg RJ. Sudden death due to cardiac arrhythmias. *New England Journal of Medicine* 2001;345:1473–82.
409 Yusuf S. *Evidence-based Cardiology*, 2nd edn. London: BMJ Books, 2003.
410 Somani P. Antiarrhythmic effects of flecainide. *Clinical Pharmacology and Therapeutics* 1980;27:464–70.

411 Moore TJ. *Deadly Medicine: Why Tens of Thousands of Heart Patients Died in America's Worst Drug Disaster.* New York: Simon & Schuster, 1995.

412 Hall N. Causation and the price of transitivity. *Journal of Philosophy* 2000;97:198–222.

413 Kvart I. Transitivity and preemption of causal relevance. *Philosophical Studies* 1991;44(125–160).

414 McDermott M. Redundant causation. *British Journal for the Philosophy of Science* 1995;46:523–44.

415 Leibovici L. Effects of remote, retroactive intercessory prayer on outcomes in patients with bloodstream infection: randomised controlled trial. *British Medical Journal* 2001;323:1450–1.

416 Schulz KF, Grimes DA. Multiplicity in randomised trials II: subgroup and interim analyses. *Lancet* 2005;365:1657–61.

417 Turk DC, Dworkin RH, McDermott MP et al. Analyzing multiple endpoints in clinical trials of pain treatments: IMMPACT recommendations. *Pain* 2008;139:485–93.

418 Pocock SJ, Hughes MD, Lee RJ. Statistical problems in the reporting of clinical trials. A survey of three medical journals. *New England Journal of Medicine* 1987;317:426–32.

419 Glennan SS. Probable causes and the distinction between subjective and objective chance. *Nous* 1997;31:496–519 (http://www.wiley.com/bw/journal.asp?ref=0029-4624).

420 Osler, Sir W. *The Principles and Practice of Medicine.* New York and London: D. Appleton and Company, 1919.

421 Spock B. *Baby and Child Care.* Illustrations by Dorothea Fox. New York: Pocket Books; London: New English Library, 1966.

422 Dwyer T, Ponsonby AL, Gibbons LE, Newman NM. Prone sleeping position and SIDS: evidence from recent case–control and cohort studies in Tasmania. *Journal of Paediatrics and Child Health* 1991;27:340–3.

423 Dwyer T, Ponsonby AL, Newman NM, Gibbons LE. Prospective cohort study of prone sleeping position and sudden infant death syndrome. *Lancet* 1991;337:1244–7.

424 Mitchell EA, Scragg R, Stewart AW et al. Results from the first year of the New Zealand cot death study. *New Zealand Medical Journal* 1991;104:71–6.

425 Gibbons LE, Ponsonby AL, Dwyer T. A comparison of prospective and retrospective responses on sudden infant death syndrome by case and control mothers. *American Journal of Epidemiology* 1993;137:654–9.

426 Irgens LM, Markestad T, Baste V, Schreuder P, Skjaerven R, Oyen N. Sleeping position and sudden infant death syndrome in Norway 1967–91. *Archives of Disease in Childhood* 1995;72:478–82.

427 Taylor JA, Krieger JW, Reay DT, Davis RL, Harruff R, Cheney LK. Prone sleep position and the sudden infant death syndrome in King County, Washington: a case–control study. *Journal of Pediatrics* 1996;128:626–30.

428 Gilbert R, Salanti G, Harden M, See S. Infant sleeping position and the sudden infant death syndrome: systematic review of observational studies and

historical review of recommendations from 1940 to 2002. *International Journal of Epidemiology* 2005;34:874–87.

429 Davies DP. Cot death in Hong Kong: a rare problem? *Lancet* 1985;ii:1346–9.

430 Lee NN, Chan YF, Davies DP, Lau E, Yip DC. Sudden infant death syndrome in Hong Kong: confirmation of low incidence. *British Medical Journal* 1989;298:721.

431 Ponsonby AL, Dwyer T, Gibbons LE, Cochrane JA, Wang YG. Factors potentiating the risk of sudden infant death syndrome associated with the prone position. *New England Journal of Medicine* 1993;329:377–82.

432 Oyen N, Haglund B, Skjaerven R, Irgens LM. Maternal smoking, birthweight and gestational age in sudden infant death syndrome (SIDS) babies and their surviving siblings. *Paediatric and Perinatal Epidemiology* 1997;11(Suppl. 1): 84–95.

433 Mitchell EA, Thompson JM, Ford RP, Taylor BJ. Sheepskin bedding and the sudden infant death syndrome. New Zealand Cot Death Study Group. *Journal of Pediatrics* 1998;133:701–4.

434 Hill AB. The environment and disease: association or causation? *Proceedings of the Royal Society of Medicine* 1965;58:295–300.

435 Fleming TR, DeMets DL. Surrogate end points in clinical trials: are we being misled? *Annals of Internal Medicine* 1996;125:605–13.

436 Prentice RL. Surrogate and mediating endpoints: current status and future directions. *Journal of the National Cancer Institute* 2009;101:216–17.

437 Prentice RL. Surrogate endpoints in clinical trials: definition and operational criteria. *Statistics in Medicine* 1989;8:431–40.

438 Johnston K. What are surrogate outcome measures and why do they fail in clinical research? *Neuroepidemiology* 1999;18:167–73.

439 Zhang B, Schmidt B. Do we measure the right end points? A systematic review of primary outcomes in recent neonatal randomized clinical trials. *Journal of Pediatrics* 2001;138:76–80.

440 De Gruttola VG, Clax P, DeMets DL et al. Considerations in the evaluation of surrogate endpoints in clinical trials. Summary of a National Institutes of Health workshop. *Controlled Clinical Trials* 2001;22:485–502.

441 Qin L, Gilbert PB, Follmann D, Li D. Assessing surrogate endpoints in vaccine trials with case-cohort sampling and the Cox model. *Annals of Applied Statistics* 2008;2:386–407.

442 Gilbert PB, Qin L, Self SG. Evaluating a surrogate endpoint at three levels, with application to vaccine development. *Statistics in Medicine* 2008;27:4758–78.

443 Kassai B, Shah NR, Leizorovicza A, Cucherat M, Gueyffier F, Boissel JP. The true treatment benefit is unpredictable in clinical trials using surrogate outcome measured with diagnostic tests. *Journal of Clinical Epidemiology* 2005;58:1042–51.

444 Expert Protein Analysis System. Metabolic Pathways. Available at www.expasy.org/cgi-bin/show_thumbnails.pl [accessed April 19, 2010]

445 Cartwright N. What is wrong with Bayes nets? *The Monist* 2001;84:242–64.

446 Hesslow G. Two notes on the probabilistic approach to causality. *Philosophy of Science* 1976;43:290–92.

447 Hauben M, Aronson JK. Paradoxical reactions: under-recognized adverse effects of drugs. *Drug Safety* 2006;29:970.

448 King T, Ossipov MH, Vanderah TW, Porreca F, Lai J. Is paradoxical pain induced by sustained opioid exposure an underlying mechanism of opioid antinociceptive tolerance? *Neurosignals* 2005;14:194–205.

449 Lai J, Ossipov MH, Vanderah TW, Malan TP Jr, Porreca F. Neuropathic pain: the paradox of dynorphin. *Molecular Interventions* 2001;1:160–7.

450 Saperia J, Ashby D, Gunnell D. Suicidal behaviour and SSRIs: updated meta-analysis. *British Medical Journal* 2006;332:1453.

451 Damluji NF, Ferguson JM. Paradoxical worsening of depressive symptomatology caused by antidepressants. *Journal of Clinical Psychopharmacology* 1988;8:347–9.

452 Gilbert SF, Sarkar S. Embracing complexity: organicism for the 21st century. *Developmental Dynamics* 2000;219:1–9.

453 Laublicher MD, Wagner GP. How molecular is molecular developmental biology? A reply to Alex Rosenberg's reductionsim redux: computing the embryo. *Biology and Philosophy* 2001;16.

454 Brigandt I, Love A. Reductionism in biology. In: Zalta EN (ed.) *The Stanford Encyclopedia of Philosophy*. Stanford, CA: Metaphysics Research Lab, Center for the Study of Language and Information, Stanford University, 2008.

455 Winkle RA, Mason JW, Griffin JC, Ross D. Malignant ventricular tachyarrhythmias associated with the use of encainide. *American Heart Journal* 1981;102:857–64.

456 Broadbent A. Causation and models of disease in epidemiology. forthcoming.

457 Nielsen VE, Bonnema SJ, Boel-Jorgensen H, Grupe P, Hegedus L. Stimulation with 0.3-mg recombinant human thyrotropin prior to iodine 131 therapy to improve the size reduction of benign nontoxic nodular goiter: a prospective randomized double-blind trial. *Archives of Internal Medicine* 2006;166: 1476–82.

458 Bonnema SJ, Nielsen VE, Boel-Jorgensen H *et al.* Improvement of goiter volume reduction after 0.3 mg recombinant human thyrotropin-stimulated radioiodine therapy in patients with a very large goiter: a double-blinded, randomized trial. *Journal of Clinical Endocrinology and Metabolism* 2007;92:3424–8.

459 Bonnema SJ, Nielsen VE, Boel-Jorgensen H *et al.* Recombinant human thyrotropin-stimulated radioiodine therapy of large nodular goiters facilitates tracheal decompression and improves inspiration. *Journal of Clinical Endocrinology and Metabolism* 2008;93:3981–4.

460 Lin YC, Chang MH, Ni YH, Hsu HY, Chen DS. Long-term immunogenicity and efficacy of universal hepatitis B virus vaccination in Taiwan. *Journal of Infectious Diseases* 2003;187:134–8.

461 McMahon BJ, Bruden DL, Petersen KM *et al.* Antibody levels and protection after hepatitis B vaccination: results of a 15-year follow-up. *Annals of Internal Medicine* 2005;142:333–41.

462   Bosnak M, Dikici B, Bosnak V, Haspolat K. Accelerated hepatitis B vaccination schedule in childhood. *Pediatrics International* 2002;44:663–5.

463   Nothdurft HD, Dietrich M, Zuckerman JN *et al*. A new accelerated vaccination schedule for rapid protection against hepatitis A and B. *Vaccine* 2002;20:1157–62.

464   Dane DS, Cameron CH, Briggs M. Virus-like particles in serum of patients with Australia-antigen-associated hepatitis. *Lancet* 1970;i:695–8.

465   Howard CR, Young PR, Lee S *et al*. Hepatitis B surface antigen polypeptide micelles from antigen expressed in *Saccharomyces cerevisiae*. *Journal of Virological Methods* 1986;14:25–35.

466   McAleer WJ, Buynak EB, Maigetter RZ, Wampler DE, Miller WJ, Hilleman MR. Human hepatitis B vaccine from recombinant yeast. *Nature* 1984;307:178–80.

467   Millman I, Eisenstein TK, Blumberg BS. *Hepatitis B the Virus, the Disease and the Vaccine*. New York: Plenum, 1984.

468   ISIS-2 (Second International Study of Infarct Survival) Collaborative Group. Randomized trial of intravenous streptokinase, oral aspirin, both, or neither among 17,187 cases of suspected acute myocardial infarction. *Lancet* 1988;ii:349–60.

469   Olshansky B, Dossey L. Retroactive prayer: a preposterous hypothesis? *British Medical Journal* 2003;327:1465–8.

470   Ohry A, Tsafrir J. Is chicken soup an essential drug? *Canadian Medical Association Journal* 1999;161:1532–3.

471   Contopoulos-Ioannidis DG, Ntzani E, Ioannidis JP. Translation of highly promising basic science research into clinical applications. *American Journal of Medicine* 2003;114:477–84.

472   Spock B. *The Pocket Book of Baby and Child Care*. Pocket Books: New York, 1956.

473   Halsted WS. I. The results of radical operations for the cure of carcinoma of the breast. *Annals of Surgery* 1907;46:1–19.

474   Allen C, Glasziou P, Del Mar C. Bed rest: a potentially harmful treatment needing more careful evaluation. *Lancet* 1999;354:1229–33.

475   Olsen O, Gøtzsche PC. Screening for breast cancer with mammography. *Cochrane Database of Systematic Reviews* 2001;(4):CD001877.

476   Olsen O, Gøtzsche PC. Cochrane review on screening for breast cancer with mammography. *Lancet* 2001;358:1340–2.

477   Hoare C, Li Wan Po A, Williams H. Systematic review of treatments for atopic eczema. *Health Technology Assessment* 2000;4(37):1–191.

478   Takwale A, Tan E, Agarwal S *et al*. Efficacy and tolerability of borage oil in adults and children with atopic eczema: randomised, double blind, placebo controlled, parallel group trial. *British Medical Journal* 2003;327:1385.

479   National Institute for Health and Clinical Excellence. Wisdom teeth removal. London: NICE, 2000.

480   Dickinson K, Roberts I. Medical anti-shock trousers (pneumatic anti-shock garments) for circulatory support in patients with trauma. *Cochrane Database of Systematic Reviews* 2000;(2):CD001856.

481 Lepor H, Williford WO, Barry MJ et al. The efficacy of terazosin, finasteride, or both in benign prostatic hyperplasia. Veterans Affairs Cooperative Studies Benign Prostatic Hyperplasia Study Group. *New England Journal of Medicine* 1996;335:533–9.

482 Meunier PJ, Sebert JL, Reginster JY et al. Fluoride salts are no better at preventing new vertebral fractures than calcium-vitamin D in postmenopausal osteoporosis: the FAVOStudy. *Osteoporosis International* 1998;8:4–12.

483 Morris JK. Screening for neuroblastoma in children. *Journal of Medical Screening* 2002;9:56.

484 Semmelweis IP. *Die Ätiologie, der Begriff und die Prophylaxis des Kindbettfiebers* (*The Etiology, Concept and Prophylaxis of Childbed Fever*). Madison: University of Wisconsin Press, 1983.

485 Marshall B. One hundred years of discovery and rediscovery of *Helicobacter pylori* and its association with peptic ulcer disease. In: Mobley HLT, Mendz GL, Hazell SL (eds) Helicobacter pylori: *Physiology and Genetics*. Washington, DC: ASM Press, 2001, chapter 3.

486 Marshall B. *Helicobacter* connections. *ChemMedChem* 2006;1:783–802.

487 Anon. Which anticonvulsant for women with eclampsia? Evidence from the Collaborative Eclampsia Trial. *Lancet* 1995;345:1455–63.

488 Englehardt HTJ. Introduction. In: Englehardt HTJ, Spicker SF, Towers B (eds) *Clinical Judgment: A Critical Appraisal*. Dordrecht: D. Reidel Publishing Company, 1977, pp. xi–xxiv.

489 Cooper JM, Hutchinson DS. *Plato. Complete Works*. Indianapolis, IN: Hackett, 1997.

490 Breart G. Documentation and use of evidence in the consensus conference proces. In: Goodman C, Baratz SR (eds) *Improving Consensus Development for Health Technology Assessment: An International Perspective*. Washington, DC: National Academy Press, 1990, pp. 23–31.

491 Ryle G. *The Concept of Mind*. Harmondsworth: Penguin Books, 1963.

492 Cochrane A, Blythe M. *One Man's Medicine*. London: The British Medical Journal, 1989.

493 Enkin M, Keirse MJ, Chalmers I. *A Guide to Effective Care in Pregnancy and Childbirth*. Oxford: Oxford University Press, 1989.

494 Crowley P, Chalmers I, Keirse MJ. The effects of corticosteroid administration before preterm delivery: an overview of the evidence from controlled trials. *British Journal of Obstetrics and Gynaecology* 1990;97:11–25.

495 NIH Consensus Development Panel on the Effect of Corticosteroids for Fetal Maturation on Perinatal Outcomes. Effect of corticosteroids for fetal maturation on perinatal outcomes. *Journal of the American Medical Association* 1995;273:413–18.

496 Reynolds LA, Tansey EM (eds) *Prenatal Corticosteroids for Reducing Morbidity and Mortality After Preterm Birth*. London: Wellcome Trust Centre, 2004.

497 Irwin F. *Letters of Thomas Jefferson*. Tilton, NH: Sanbornton Bridge Press, 1975.

498 Cochrane JA. *Effectiveness and Efficiency: Random Reflections on Health Services*. London: Nuffield Provincial Hospitals Trust, 1972.

499 Bonadonna G, Valagussa P, Moliterni A, Zambetti M, Brambilla C. Adjuvant cyclophosphamide, methotrexate, and fluorouracil in node-positive breast cancer: the results of 20 years of follow-up. *New England Journal of Medicine* 1995;332:901–6.

500 Branthwaite A, Cooper P. Analgesic effects of branding in treatment of headaches. *British Medical Journal* 1981;282:1576–8.

501 Waber RL, Shiv B, Carmon Z, Ariely D. Commercial features of placebo and therapeutic efficacy. *Journal of the American Medical Association* 2008;299:1016–17.

502 Pollo A, Amanzio M, Casadio C, Maggi G, Benedetti F. Response expectancies in placebo analgesia and their clinical relevance. *Pain* 2001;93:77–84.

503 Tversky A, Kahneman D. Judgment under uncertainty: heuristics and biases. *Science* 1974;185:1124–31.

504 Gigerenzer G. *Reckoning with Risk: Learning to Live with Uncertainty*. London: Penguin, 2003.

505 Sober E. The art and science of clinical judgment. In: Englehardt HTJ, Spicker SF, Towers B (eds) *Clinical Judgment: A Critical Appraisal*. Dordrecht: D. Reidel Publishing Company, 1977, pp. 29–44.

506 Rothwell PM. Can overall results of clinical trials be applied to all patients? *Lancet* 1995;345:1616–19.

507 Dawes RM, Faust D, Meehl PE. Clinical versus actuarial judgment. *Science* 1989;243:1668–74.

508 Scriven M. Clinical judgment. In: Englehardt HTJ, Spicker SF, Towers B (eds) *Clinical Judgment: A Critical Appraisal*. Dordrecht: D. Reidel Publishing Company, 1977.

509 Meehl PE. *Clinical Versus Statistical Prediction: A Theoretical Analysis and a Review of the Evidence*. Minneapolis: University of Minnesota Press, 1996.

510 de Dombal FT, Leaper DJ, Staniland JR, McCann AP, Horrocks JC. Computer-aided diagnosis of acute abdominal pain. *British Medical Journal* 1972;2:9–13.

511 Gough HG. Clinical versus statistical prediction in psychology. In: Postman L (ed.) *Psychology in the Making*. New York: Knopf, 1962.

512 Sawyer J. Measurement and prediction, clinical and statistical. *Psychological Bulletin* 1966;66:178–200.

513 Dawes RM. How clinical probability judgments may be used to validate diagnostic signs. *Journal of Clinical Psychology* 1967;23:403–10.

514 Grove WM, Zald DH, Lebow BS, Snitz BE, Nelson C. Clinical versus mechanical prediction: a meta-analysis. *Psychological Assessment* 2000;12:19–30.

515 McReynolds P (ed.) *Advances in Psychological Assessment*. Palo Alto, CA: Science and Behavior Books, 1968.

516 Holt RR. Clinical and statistical prediction: a reformulation and some new data. *Journal of Abnormal Psychology* 1958;56:1–12.

517 Holt RR. Yet another look at clinical and statistical prediction: or, is clinical psychology worthwhile? *American Psychologist* 1970;25:337–49.

518 Choudhry NK, Fletcher RH, Soumerai SB. Systematic review: the relationship between clinical experience and quality of health care. *Annals of Internal Medicine* 2005;142:260–73.

519 Kruger J, Dunning D. Unskilled and unaware of it: how difficulties in recognizing one's own incompetence lead to inflated self-assessments. *Journal of Personality and Social Psychology* 1999;77:1121–34.

520 Cannon SR, Gardner RM. Experience with a computerized interactive protocol system using HELP. *Computers and Biomedical Research* 1980;13:399–409.

521 Bachmann LM, Kolb E, Koller MT, Steurer J, ter Riet G. Accuracy of Ottawa ankle rules to exclude fractures of the ankle and mid-foot: systematic review. *British Medical Journal* 2003;326:417.

522 Stiell IG, Greenberg GH, McKnight RD, Nair RC, McDowell I, Worthington JR. A study to develop clinical decision rules for the use of radiography in acute ankle injuries. *Annals of Emergency Medicine* 1992;21:384–90.

523 Stiell IG, Wells GA, Hoag RH *et al*. Implementation of the Ottawa Knee Rule for the use of radiography in acute knee injuries. *Journal of the American Medical Association* 1997;278:2075–9.

524 Knaus WA, Draper EA, Wagner DP, Zimmerman JE. APACHE II: a severity of disease classification system. *Critical Care Medicine* 1985;13:818–29.

525 McGinn TG, Guyatt GH, Wyer PC, Naylor CD, Stiell IG, Richardson WS. Users' guides to the medical literature: XXII: how to use articles about clinical decision rules. *Journal of the American Medical Association* 2000;284: 79–84.

526 Wasson JH, Sox HC, Neff RK, Goldman L. Clinical prediction rules. Applications and methodological standards. *New England Journal of Medicine* 1985;313:793–9.

527 Meehl PE. Causes and effects of my disturbing little book. *Journal of Personality Assessment* 1986;50:370–5.

528 Greenhalgh T. Bayesian decision making in primary care or how to stop people dying of chicken pox. *Trials and Tribulations—Evidence, Medical Decision-Making and Policy* 2008.

529 Horrocks JC, McCann AP, Staniland JR, Leaper DJ, De Dombal FT. Computer-aided diagnosis: description of an adaptable system, and operational experience with 2,034 cases. *British Medical Journal* 1972;2:5–9.

530 British Medical Association. Quality and Outcomes Framework guidance for GMS contract 2009/10. Delivering investment in general practice. London: BMA, 2009.

531 Deveugele M, Derese A, van den Brink-Muinen A, Bensing J, De Maeseneer J. Consultation length in general practice: cross sectional study in six European countries. *British Medical Journal* 2002;325:472.

532 Lown B. *The Lost Art of Healing*. Boston: Houghton Mifflin, 1996.

533 Birch S. Which are the placebo effects: comment on Kaptchuk *et al.*'s IBS placebo study. Available at www.bmj.com/letters/ [accessed June 30, 2008]

534 Polanyi M. *Personal Knowledge. Towards a Post-critical Philosophy*. London: Routledge and Kegan Paul, 1958.

535 Thornton T. Tacit knowledge as the unifying factor in evidence based medicine and clinical judgement. *Philosophy, Ethics and Humanities in Medicine* 2006;1:E2.

536 Bero L, Oostvogel F, Bacchetti P, Lee K. Factors associated with findings of published trials of drug–drug comparisons: why some statins appear more efficacious than others. *PLoS Med* 2007;4(6):e184.

537 Jorgensen AW, Hilden J, Gøtzsche PC. Cochrane reviews compared with industry supported meta-analyses and other meta-analyses of the same drugs: systematic review. *British Medical Journal* 2006;333:782.

538 Leopold SS, Warme WJ, Fritz Braunlich E, Shott S. Association between funding source and study outcome in orthopaedic research. *Clinical Orthopaedics and Related Research* 2003;(415):293–301.

539 Lexchin J, Bero LA, Djulbegovic B, Clark O. Pharmaceutical industry sponsorship and research outcome and quality: systematic review. *British Medical Journal* 2003;326:1167–70.

540 Yaphe J, Edman R, Knishkowy B, Herman J. The association between funding by commercial interests and study outcome in randomized controlled drug trials. *Family Practice* 2001;18:565–8.

541 Heres S, Davis J, Maino K, Jetzinger E, Kissling W, Leucht S. Why olanzapine beats risperidone, risperidone beats quetiapine, and quetiapine beats olanzapine: an exploratory analysis of head-to-head comparison studies of second-generation antipsychotics. *American Journal of Psychiatry* 2006;163:185–94.

542 Smith R. Medical journals are an extension of the marketing arm of pharmaceutical companies. *PLoS Med* 2005;2(5):e138.

543 Hopewell S, Loudon K, Clarke MJ, Oxman AD, Dickersin K. Publication bias in clinical trials due to statistical significance or direction of trial results. *Cochrane Database of Systematic Reviews* 2009;(1):MR000006.

544 Turner EH, Matthews AM, Linardatos E, Tell RA, Rosenthal R. Selective publication of antidepressant trials and its influence on apparent efficacy. *New England Journal of Medicine* 2008;358:252–60.

545 De Angelis C, Drazen JM, Frizelle FA *et al.* Clinical trial registration: a statement from the International Committee of Medical Journal Editors. *New England Journal of Medicine* 2004;351:1250–1.

546 Tramer MR, Reynolds DJ, Moore RA, McQuay HJ. Impact of covert duplicate publication on meta-analysis: a case study. *British Medical Journal* 1997;315:635–40.

547 Gøtzsche P. Bias in double-blind trials [thesis]. *Danish Medical Bulletin* 1990;37:329–36.

548 Gøtzsche PC. Methodology and overt and hidden bias in reports of 196 double-blind trials of nonsteroidal antiinflammatory drugs in rheumatoid arthritis. *Controlled Clinical Trials* 1989;10:31–56.

549 Gøtzsche PC. Blinding during data analysis and writing of manuscripts. *Controlled Clinical Trials* 1996;17:285–90; discussion 90–3.

550 Stelfox HT, Chua G, O'Rourke K, Detsky AS. Conflict of interest in the debate over calcium-channel antagonists. *New England Journal of Medicine* 1998;338:101–6.

551 Wilkinson R, Marmot M (eds) *Social Determinants of Health: The Solid Facts*, 2nd edn. Copenhagen: World Health Organization, 2003.

Index

Printed and bound by CPI Group (UK) Ltd, Croydon, CR0 4YY

Printed and bound by CPI Group (UK) Ltd, Croydon, CR0 4YY

27/10/2024

14580383-0001